Medicine in Wales, c.1800–2000

Medicine in Wales
c.1800–2000

PUBLIC SERVICE OR PRIVATE COMMODITY?

edited by

ANNE BORSAY

*Published on behalf of the History and Law Committee of the
Board of Celtic Studies of the University of Wales*

UNIVERSITY OF WALES PRESS
CARDIFF
2003

British Library Cataloguing-in-Publication Data.
A catalogue record for this book is available from the British Library.

ISBN 0–7083–1824–X

Typeset by Bryan Turnbull
Printed in Great Britain by Dinefwr Press, Llandybïe

Contents

ॐ

Acknowledgements

◆

This volume arose from a meeting in 1999 at the University of Wales Conference Centre, Gregynog on the theme, 'Public/Private: Multi-disciplinary Perspectives on Medicine and Health in Wales'. The editor and contributors are grateful to the inter-collegiate Staff Colloquia Fund and the Wellcome Trust for their generous support of this gathering. Publication has been funded by the Board of Celtic Studies, to whom we also express our thanks. We have benefited greatly from the comments of the Board's anonymous referee and from the support of Dr Paul O'Leary in his capacity as secretary of the History and Law Committee.

Anne Borsay

List of Illustrations

ॐ

List of Contributors

෨

Anne Borsay B.Sc.Econ. (Wales), M.Litt. (Oxon), Ph.D. (Wales) is a professor in the School of Health Science at the University of Wales Swansea.

Sara Brady BA (Bath Spa University College), MA (Wales) is a part-time Ph.D. student in the Department of History at the University of Wales, Lampeter. She also works in Information Services at Cardiff University.

Richard Coopey MA, Ph.D. (Warwick), FRSA is a lecturer in economic history at the University of Wales, Aberystwyth and a senior research fellow at the London School of Economics. He is president of the International Water History Association.

Mark Drakeford BA (Kent), B.Phil. (Exeter), Ph.D. (Wales), CQSW teaches at Cardiff University and is currently on secondment to the Welsh Assembly, where he is a policy adviser to the health minister.

David Greaves MB, BS, MA (London), M.Litt. (Aberdeen), Ph.D. (Wales) is an honorary senior lecturer in medical humanities at the University of Wales Swansea.

David Hirst B.Sc.Soc. (London), MA (Manchester), Ph.D. (Wales) is a senior lecturer in social policy at the University of Wales, Bangor.

Pamela Michael BA, MA, Ph.D. (Wales) is a lecturer in health and social policy at the University of Wales, Bangor.

Susan J. Pitt, BA, Ph.D. (Wales) was awarded her doctorate by the University of Wales, Lampeter in 1996.

Dorothy Porter BA, MA (Sussex), Ph.D. (London) is a professor in the Department of Anthropology, History and Social Medicine at the University of California, San Francisco.

Owen Roberts BA (York) is a lecturer in history at the University of Wales, Aberystwyth.

Steven Thompson BA, Ph.D. (Wales) is a lecturer in history at the University of Wales, Aberystwyth.

Anthea Symonds B.Sc. (Bath), M.Sc. (Sussex), Ph.D. (Birmingham) is a part-time lecturer in social policy at the University of Wales Swansea.

1

Medicine and Health: Historical and Contemporary Perspectives

ഔ

ANNE BORSAY and DOROTHY PORTER

Introduction

In the past thirty years, the historical study of medicine and health has undergone a revolution. From origins in the celebration of great medical men and their clinical achievements, it has tapped into social and cultural history, and pulled in concepts from the social sciences, to become a seedbed for interdisciplinary research.[1] Welsh historiography has been slow to respond to this new subdiscipline. Most research is contained in MA, M.Phil or Ph.D. theses and published work is typically written in the heroic or antiquarian tradition. The reasons for this time lag are bound up with the rapid industrialization of the south Wales coalfield post-1870 and the trauma of its economic decline after the First World War. Histories produced in the early twentieth century were largely indifferent to this industrial past, privileging instead a more distant and uniformly rural heritage. By 1950 the economic history of the coalfield was being written, and during the 1960s this brief was extended to include the radical labour and political relations of the Valleys. The effect has been a split within Welsh historiography which has marginalized the rural – and often Welsh-speaking – areas, and led to a neglect of many aspects of social history.[2] More than a decade ago, Deian Hopkin argued that there were 'far too many empty shelves, where studies of demography, migration, standards of living, patterns of consumption, health, welfare and education should sit'.[3] His conclusion is still valid today.

This collection of essays is a contribution to the social history of medicine and health in Wales. Compiled to illustrate the growing corpus of research-based material, its content is deliberately diverse. No one theoretical position prevails, and a wide variety of sources are drawn on which range beyond the historians' staple diet of documentary records to film, oral testimony, and participatory social research. To ensure coherence, however, each chapter is located within its general intellectual context, and this introduction sets out a conceptual framework for the debates which revolve around medicine and health at the opening of the twenty-first century.

Modernity and Enlightenment

Our contemporary experiences of medicine and health are bound up with the trajectory of modernity. Political historians tend to date this era from the French Revolution of 1789, a cataclysmic event that sent shock waves across Europe. Social and cultural historians, on the other hand, associate it with the Enlightenment or the age of reason. In the past, a preoccupation with the great French-speaking philosophers has traced the Enlightenment to the early eighteenth century. The British Isles, however, were showing signs of this mentality from the seventeenth century: in the constitutional arrangements which followed the 'Glorious Revolution' of 1688; in the toleration of religious Dissenters, linked to these; and, critically for medicine, in the scientific revolution which was exemplified by William Harvey's investigations into the circulation of the blood published in 1628. The ideas that underpinned these changes situated all human suffering in ignorance and superstition, and insisted that scientific knowledge would lead to human progress without limit. As a consequence, observation and experiment were favoured over the a priori reasoning which had characterized both the classical Renaissance and the Protestant Reformation; the automatic acceptance of traditional knowledge was challenged, releasing humanity from the condemnation of original sin; and secular sciences of man were promoted to inform strategies for personal, social and political improvement.[4]

The application of this Enlightenment thinking was aided by a flourishing capitalist economy and a strong nation-state of which

Wales was a part. Though variable in its geographical impact, expanding trade and commerce produced wealth which spread to the urban middling sort well before the Industrial Revolution turned Victorian Britain into the workshop of the world.[5] The resources generated by this economic base were initially channelled into voluntary schemes of improvement. The prospering classes not only civilized themselves through the support of uplifting cultural activities, but also tried to better the lower orders by funding a series of charitable endeavours which included hospitals and dispensaries.[6] During the course of the nineteenth century, these 'private' initiatives were joined by 'public' policies. Previously active in pursuing commercial interests abroad, the nation-state slowly cast off its residual role in home affairs.[7] More collective responsibility was assumed for the quality of the environment[8] and for the physical and mental health of the people,[9] whose rights as citizens were being enhanced through a gradual extension of the parliamentary franchise.[10] Decline relative to foreign competitors from the 1870s, and the Depression of the 1930s, dented confidence in modernity's economic agenda,[11] and the political credentials of all nation-states were undermined by the atrocities of fascism and communism, and by the carnage of the First and Second World Wars. Yet despite these setbacks, the Enlightenment commitment to rationalism and progress proved resilient, and by the late 1940s Britain exemplified a modern society at the pinnacle of its development.

Public Health and Private Lives

A defining feature of this modernity was the welfare state and the commitment to public health care that it embodied. The historiography of welfare states has previously conceptualized them as comprehensive systems of social security, funded and administered by the centralized political organizations which emerged in northern Europe during the first half of the nineteenth century.[12] More recent studies, however, have begun to explore the changing forms of welfare provided by a myriad of agencies, from self-help and mutual aid to various types of collective distribution arranged by political, voluntaristic or commercial institutions, in communities with or without a centralization of power.[13] This approach has highlighted the way in which distinctions between the private and the public delivery of health care became blurred. For medicine, an important aspect of the process has been the concentration upon private lives by public health practice, brought about by the academic discipline of social medicine that was institutionalized in British universities during and immediately after the Second World War.[14] Gone were the sewers and drains of public health policy, and the eugenically tainted strategies for social hygiene pursued in respect of physical and mental deficiency. And in their place was put a new science of socio-medical reform, which married the genetic basis of health with the social demographic analysis of disease, and then applied the outcome of this synthesis to the evaluation of health care. Social medicine was therefore an expression of the Enlightenment mission to create a utopia of reason.

This visionary notion of social medicine resonated with the political spirit of the age: the mid-twentieth-century revulsion against fascism in the Western democracies which propelled intellectuals towards scientific rationalism as the means to construct a just and equal society in accordance with their socialist convictions. By the late 1950s, however, the grand view of social medicine as political action was diminishing under the influence of a narrow quantification, which was in turn reinforced by the success of epidemiology in identifying tobacco smoking as the main cause of lung cancer. Such positivism was not regarded as incompatible with the socialist aspirations of social medicine because objective scientific facts were seen as the building blocks of the new society. None the less, there was an increasing pre-occupation with the relationships between health, illness and social behaviour rather than with the social structural determinants of health, and the emphasis shifted to the reformation of individual lifestyles rather than the abolition of inequality.

Interlocking with the evolution of social medicine were key demographic and epidemiological transitions which produced an ageing and hence more chronically sick population. Therefore, the promotion of healthy lifestyles became an attractive rearguard action to reduce the rising costs of medical services. Under this scenario, individuals were construed as responsible for their health behaviour by public information campaigns which sought to raise consciousness, encourage self-care, and so prevent a wide variety of chronic conditions – cardio-vascular disorders, digestive complaints, venereal diseases, obesity and stress, as well as the smoking-related illnesses with which the strategy originated. There have been two significant effects: the creation of a 'worried-well' society where everybody perceives themselves as potential patients;[15] and the stigmatization of the diseased by blaming them for their illnesses. The campaigns to prevent chronic illness through individual diet and exercise spread fear of the consequences of failing to live a healthy lifestyle. Levels of anxiety among the well have been reflected in the massive growth in the commercialization of health aids, dietary regimes, and what can only be described as an exercise industry. In the late twentieth century, the healthy body produced by a healthy lifestyle created a new moral map of social citizenship by becoming not only one of the qualifications for membership of the cosmopolitan elite, but also a moral instruction to the powerless and economically disadvantaged that achieving health, beauty and desirability is a social duty.

This message has been reinforced by the moral disgust bestowed on the diseased, broken, abused, self-indulged or neglected body, and by the blame assigned to patients for their own disorders. Recent advertisements for the British Heart Foundation stigmatize the thrombotic heart patient as an ignorant, lazy, high-fat-eating, beer-swilling, cigarette-smoking working-class lout, who recognizes too late his duty to his family to keep well. Public health campaigns against lung cancer, liver disease and venereal infection have pictured the sick as similar social pariahs, failures, moral inferiors, reprobates, and inadequates. Paradoxically, however, the individualistic emphasis of the new social contract between the modern state and its citizens allows the right to consume to remain a priority. The obligation to be healthy continues to be subordinate to the right of every citizen in a free-market democracy to be a consumer. Thus the lack of legal prohibition on the sale of tobacco serves the state's claim that *ill health*, like health, is an individual liberty: a personal choice which the state interferes with less and less in order to reduce the costs of public intervention. Therefore, those who are identified as choosing ill health face the consequences with ever-diminishing state assistance. Private health insurance for cigarette smokers has high premiums, but is increasingly necessary because smokers find it harder and harder to be treated by state-provided services. The first heavy smokers to be refused treatment by the National Health Service made headline news; now such practices are becoming standard.

From Modernity to Postmodernity?

The privatization of public health is part of a more general challenge to the classic welfare state which is no longer celebrated as the means by which to plan a guaranteed minimum level of income, education, housing and health for every citizen. Other modernist assumptions have also been undermined: the capacity of government intervention to put the public interest above private profits in a free-market economy; the organization of social relations around the structure of capitalism, with the working class at the bottom of a hierarchical ladder and women's paid labour subordinated to their domestic duties; the efficacy of nominal political equality through universal suffrage within a system of parliamentary democracy. Behind this questioning was a welfare state failing to deliver health and social care, an economy in ongoing crisis, and political institutions and procedures that were losing credibility. The apparent disintegration of the modernity project has been accompanied by profound new developments. The autonomy of the nation-state is being eroded by economic globalization, and by information and communication technologies which are also allowing flexibility at the workplace. Personal identities are becoming more fragmented as ascription by class and gender weakens, and the consumption of goods and services takes on greater significance. And power is becoming more fluid as political loyalties are constructed around lifestyles, regions or particular issues, rather than determined by fixed party allegiances. At the core of modernity's predicament, however, is a loss of faith in the rationalism of the Enlightenment and the planned society managed by experts which represented the culmination of this mentality in the second half of the twentieth century.[16]

Though the gravity of these changes has led some historians and sociologists to contend that a new era of postmodernity has dawned, assaults on modernity are not without precedent. After all, Marx berated the exploitation of the capitalist economic system and the resulting alienation of workers. Durkheim pointed to the disintegrative effects of a rigid division of labour. And Weber 'feared that rationalization would eventually crush the human spirit, walling it in behind the bars of the bureaucratic iron cage'.[17] However, it was the Critical Theory of the Frankfurt School that in the 1930s first called into question the Enlightenment adherence to reason. Seeing rationalization as the 'essence' of Western civilization, they argued that it was inherently repressive. Science and philosophy were 'part of the fabric of capitalist society', which 'sustain[ed] its ideals under the guise of pure, disinterested, objective inquiry'. Therefore, 'Only a critical theory that unmask[ed] these connections . . . [could] provide a way of criticizing modern capitalist culture and retrieve the Enlightenment connections between knowledge and emancipation from exploitation, ideology and power.'[18] Postmodernism has taken this analysis further. 'We should admit', wrote Michel Foucault, 'that power produces knowledge, that power and knowledge directly imply one another; that there is no power relation without the correlative constitution of a field of knowledge, nor any knowledge that does not presuppose and constitute at the same time power relations.'[19] Any hope of rescuing the old order is thus abandoned because politics unavoidably pollute rationality. As Jean-François Lyotard – perhaps modernity's most scathing critic – emotively asks: 'What kind of thought is able to sublate Auschwitz in a general (either empirical or speculative) process towards universal emancipation?'[20]

The politicization of rationality has profound repercussions for medicine and health because notions of professional practice have previously rested on the command of discrete bodies of (largely unchallenged) expertise. Boundaries collapse as different employment groups battle for supremacy. The lay knowledge – possessed by the consumers of services, their relatives, friends, and neighbours – enjoys enhanced status. And with these shifts in the traditional balances of power comes a fragmentation of personal and professional identities, formerly fixed around not just occupation but also class, gender, community and nation. The rational individuals of Enlightenment thought thus dissolve into human subjects, faced with the prospect of reflexively constructing self-identities by 'sustaining . . . coherent, yet continuously revised, biographical narratives'.[21] Whilst postmodernists delight in the disappearance of economic, social and political structures, their critics worry that these divisions are merely concealed by a charade of consumer choice which disadvantages both the many, less powerful producers of health care and those who use their services. In search for a defence of besieged rationality, scholars have turned to the German philosopher, Jürgen Habermas. Born in 1929, Habermas was an heir to the early Frankfurt School.[22] He accused critical theory and postmodernism alike of undue pessimism, and he represented modernity as an unfinished rather than a dead project, still capable of rescue from an absolute relativity of knowledge and its attendant perils. Furthermore, his notion of the 'public sphere' offered fertile opportunities for critiquing the deconstructed welfare state.

Habermas and the Public Sphere

Although Habermas first set out his ideas on the 'public sphere' in 1962, it was not until 1989 that an English-language edition of this work, entitled *The Structural Transformation of the Public Sphere: An Inquiry into a Category of Bourgeois Society*, was published.[23] In a study that combined materials and methods from sociology and economics, law and political science, social and cultural history, Habermas embarked upon a definition and description of the historically specific 'public sphere' in early modern Britain, France and Germany.[24] In his interpretation, the creation and development of the 'public sphere' arose from the clash between an emergent bourgeoisie and the ancient, absolute monarchy. Along with the 'private sphere' which dealt in 'commitment', this 'public sphere' of 'influence' constituted what Habermas called the 'life-world', in contrast to the 'system' which comprised the economy producing 'money' and the state producing 'power'. Civil society was the intermediary: a collection of 'more or less spontaneously emergent associations, organizations and movements that, attuned to how societal problems resonate in the private life spheres, distil and transmit such reactions in amplified form to the public sphere'.[25] The outcome was a space where matters of general interest and concern were discussed in a rational and critical manner by private people coming together through the public use of their reason.[26] Both the quality of discourse and the degree of popular participation were crucial because the existence of a 'public sphere' depended upon the merits of the arguments and not the status of their proponents.[27]

Habermas believed that the bourgeois 'public sphere' did not survive the modern period, being eroded and finally destroyed by the mutual infiltration of the state and civil society: 'That society was essentially a private sphere became questionable . . . when the powers of 'society' themselves assumed functions of public authority.'[28] With this destruction of its intrinsic elements, the bourgeois 'public sphere' was left as an area within which conflicting interests competed against each other in order to achieve their aims. Organizations and pressure groups representing diverse and often narrow constituencies bargained and compromised with each other and the government, whilst denying the public access to this decision-making process. Though public opinion was still important, it did not take the shape of rational debate as previously, but degenerated into plebiscitary acclamation for the conclusions reached and implemented. Therefore the media were less a medium for discussion and criticism than a means of managing consensus,[29] as the public was transformed from a 'culture-debating' to a 'culture-consuming' corps.[30]

Yet despite this historical analysis, Habermas has more recently insisted that an expansion of the 'public sphere' is capable of breaking modernity's political impasse. 'From the perspective of democratic theory,' he argued in 1996, 'the public sphere must . . . not only detect and identify problems but also convincingly and *influentially* thematize them, furnish them with possible solutions, and dramatize them in such a way that they are taken up and dealt with by parliamentary complexes.'[31] For this to happen, however, 'subject-centred reason' had to be compromised. Consequently, the autonomous individuals of modernist discourse were rejected, and their free agency subordinated to a 'communicative rationality' or interaction in which consensus was arrived at through negotiation between equals directed towards resisting further bureaucratic intrusion into the lifeworld; in search of an 'ideal speech situation', the 'Barriers to free and open communication . . . [were to] be dismantled.'[32] The chapters that follow explore these issues with reference to medicine and health in Wales between 1800 and 2000, paying particular attention to the impact of rationality, the modern state, class and gender.

Rationality and the Modern State

For Habermas, the growing power of the state spelt the collapse of a bourgeois 'public sphere' where private individuals could exercise rationality in political affairs. However, state expansion was itself predicated upon rational discourses that became the currency of a proliferating professional army. Therefore, as Richard Coopey and Owen Roberts point out in chapter 2, the municipalization of the water supply was from the 1860s framed in terms of a series of public health arguments; namely, that competition was wasteful, and failed to deliver sufficient water of good quality to poorer and non-corporate consumers. The municipal authorities also sought expert opinion to justify their preference for upland water, in the same way that the private companies turned to rival specialists willing to argue that deep wells yielded a purer product. Coopey and Roberts insist nevertheless that the progressive, heroic historiography of state intervention has to be revised. Not only did many private companies in Wales continue to supply their customers with satisfactory water but, far from being beaten into action by a central government with new powers, local authorities took the initiative under the influence of political factors. In municipal water schemes, therefore, scientific knowledge jostled with civic pride and civic politics, as English cities colonized Wales through the erection of impressive infrastructures that were the outcome of self-interested transactions between local politicians and industrialists intent on consolidating their financial power.

Disputed professional expertise also infused that most intimate of lifeworld problems, suicide. Pamela Michael demonstrates in chapter 3 how this extreme form of private, communicative action caught the public imagination. Initially translated into the public domain through the popular culture of folklore, ballads and newspapers, suicide from the mid-nineteenth century was absorbed into a scientific discourse of medicine, sociology and psychology which, despite being contested, gradually overthrew lay interpretations. Recognizing that a Welsh-speaking facility was vital to the treatment of all mental illnesses in north Wales, doctors collaborated with charitable subscribers and local magistrates to establish a public asylum at Denbigh. In its turn, the asylum compiled a suicide narrative, using the annual reports to portray the image of a caring institution, worthy of assuming the rational management of a condition previously contained within the 'private spheres' of relatives, friends and neighbours.

The family, displaced from handling suicides, was active in filtering the interventions of the School Medical Service after its introduction in 1907. Writing in chapter 4, David Hirst investigates the impact of the service upon Welsh children, whether in rural areas or in the urban areas at whose problems the legislation was specifically aimed. He suggests that although children were now regarded as public assets with productive and reproductive potential, the relationship between the family and the state was unresolved. Some parents objected to the public spectacle of medical examination, particularly for older girls whose decency was seen as in jeopardy. However, the Board of Education was also ambivalent about the care of conditions uncovered by inspection, anxious neither to threaten the viability of private and charitable medicine nor to pauperize families by undermining their duty to meet the medical needs of their children. The failure of private self-help schemes, and a growing awareness that school clinics responded to ailments that would not be adequately managed by hospitals or private practitioners, encouraged the expansion of public provision in the years leading up to 1914, with local education authorities often waiving the legal requirement to charge for treatment.

Health policy during the inter-war period was characterized more by consolidation than innovation. During the Second World War, however, the Emergency Medical Service built on the partnerships between the public and private sectors which had been developing since the nineteenth century to offer a comprehensive strategy for meeting the needs of the conflict. This fusion prepared fertile soil for the post-war welfare state. The vision of social medicine promoted so enthusiastically at this time did not fully materialize, but from 1948 hospitals and general practice as well as the varied work of local authority health departments (which were offering embryonic community services in addition to environmental monitoring) came under state control. Even water was nationalized, although the ten multi-purpose authorities that the Thatcher government was to transfer to private ownership did not come into being until 1973. Therefore, though the water industry fell outside the National Health Service, its privatization in 1989 breached a collectivist spirit which had prevailed for hundred years.

The commodification of a good long regarded as a suitable candidate for public ownership was implemented by a Conservative government, ideologically committed to rolling back the frontiers of the state. Though a regulatory body was put in place, its priority was the profitability of the privatized companies. Mark Drakeford's evaluation in chapter 10 shows that this objective was incompatible with customer interests. Water became increasingly expensive, charges were subject to regional variation, and the social security benefits upon which poorer users relied were sensitive to neither these differences nor to the extra costs incurred by chronically sick and disabled people with special needs. Equally disturbing were the arrangements for debt collection and disconnection. In parallel with economic privatization, the companies – and Dŵr Cymru in particular – engaged in a process of social privatization which relocated with the private sector individual obligations which the public sector had formerly assumed. Elected in 1997, New Labour moved to make the protection of customer interests the primary duty of the regulator. The invidious prepayment meters, which had led a high proportion of poorer users to disconnect themselves due to financial pressure, were also banned. However, this attempt at applying state control to private ownership has yet to convince that the market system is capable of liberating consumers and delivering them desirable public goods.

The regulation of water, mental health, and child welfare all involved the implementation of state policies via different central–local matrices that were then mediated by individual users and those who played a significant role in their access to services. Habermas's public/private dichotomy inadequately captures these subtle relations. The debate about water focused on the statutory/commercial interface, whereas the Denbigh asylum was the outcome of a statutory/voluntary alliance, and the School Medical Service – a local authority provision – was anxious not to impinge upon charitable and commercial facilities. Yet none of these complexities are accommodated in a 'public sphere' confined to bourgeois opinion and a 'private sphere' that fails to distinguish profit-making enterprises from voluntary endeavours and the activities of families and communities. Therefore, Habermas's dichotomy is better replaced by the concept of a mixed economy in which the public or state sector and the private or commercial sector are conceived as separate from the charitable or voluntary sector and the informal sector comprising relatives, friends and neighbours.

Class and Gender

As well as oversimplifying the configuration of 'public' and 'private', Habermas also overlooked the effects of class and gender. Before the welfare state, the medical aid societies of south Wales offered hospital care, and domiciliary and industrial nursing, on the principle of mutuality, to a large proportion of local workmen and their families. As Steven Thompson shows in chapter 5, these societies afforded their members the chance to engage in lively debate grounded in an experiential knowledge of local conditions and services. The levels of participatory democracy and informed discourse that were achieved merit their designation as a proletarian 'public sphere'. Moreover, whilst attitudes to the inclusion of employers were divided, there was unity in attacking doctors who extracted exorbitant fees or reacted negatively to medical needs which were often defined from the perspective of the patient. An alternative world-view of public service was therefore propounded, expressing a working-class identity based on the ideals of organized labour.

If the medical aid societies discredit the idea of an exclusively bourgeois 'public sphere', Anne Borsay's look at the treatment of industrial accidents in chapter 7 indicates that such independence may have had difficulty in thriving when the state became more interventionist during the Second World War. In 1944, the Caerphilly District Miners' Hospital and the Talygarn Rehabilitation Centre, two institutions serving the south Wales coalfield that were closely associated with the trade union movement, were featured in the official film magazine, *Worker and War-Front*. The film-makers who produced the documentary believed that their new medium was a way of extending the 'public sphere' to the working class, and the footage was indeed shown to big audiences at factory and social venues. Far from stimulating critical debate, however, the images which were conveyed patronized their viewers. The homely family care of injured workers was denigrated; the professional skills of rehabilitation staff were exalted; patients were subordinated to this expertise; and those who could not be 'mended' were marginalized through the coupling of citizenship and employment. Furthermore, these negative messages were echoed by the journal of the South Wales Miners' Federation. In sharp contrast to the assurance of the medical aid societies, the economic logic of war was undermining the working-class identity which before 1939 had infused health care in the Valleys.

In representing industrial rehabilitation, the documentary film traded in stereotypes of masculinity and femininity to emphasize the strength and the vulnerability of the miner within a rigid sexual division of labour. Outside this imagery, gender relations were more nuanced, as the professional lives of nurses, midwives and health visitors illustrate. In chapter 6, Sara Brady unpicks the tradition of public service in nursing, and its preoccupation with private self-sacrifice in the name of the patient. Taking the King Edward VII Hospital (later known as the Cardiff Royal Infirmary) as a case study, she maintains that probationers training during the First World War were motivated not only by the prospect of 'doing good' but also by the social and professional rewards on offer. Predominantly from middle-class backgrounds, these women were keen to distance themselves both from working-class nurses whose occupational roots were in housewifery and from the Voluntary Aid Detachments who were often socially superior but of amateur status. The resolution of these tensions was pursued by qualifying at a prestigious institution like the King Edward VII, and by acquiring specialist knowledge and gaining promotion. The hospital faced serious cash crises between 1914 and 1918, as voluntary donations and subscriptions lagged behind expenditure, and government compensation for the additional costs of treating military patients proved insufficient. However, staff were a valued resource to be retained in a market rendered more competitive by wartime shortages and exciting opportunities to work abroad. Therefore, the management committee was sympathetic to the private ambitions of its female staff, and responded with increased wages and training in state-of-the-art skills like massage and electrical treatment. Under these circumstances, nurses were able to construct professional identities in which altruism and personal interest combined.

If nursing was a career in the making for women during the First World War, the gendered connotations of their traverse from the private, feminine domain of domesticity to the public, masculine domain of medicine were complex. In chapter 8, Susan Pitt explores childbirth in Swansea between 1948 and 1974, using oral-history interviews with doctors and midwives, and evidence from medical and midwifery textbooks.[33] She argues that there was no simple equation between gender and the public/private dichotomy because both spheres underwent a process of masculinization. In the 'public sphere', changing conceptions of district and community led to a weakening of the autonomous role of the peripatetic midwife as the hospital consultant became the central figure. In the 'private sphere', woman-to-woman relationships between the extended family and female neighbours were eroded as the nuclear family became the basic unit of society, and the father entered the delivery room. Additionally, developments in techniques of visualization during pregnancy and monitoring during labour meant that the birthing woman's body was no longer private, but violated by the masculine desire to know that was one of the defining characteristics of public medical discourse. It is concluded that this masculinization was the cause of the discomfort which led many women to complain about their experience of childbirth in the 1970s and 1980s.

Anthea Symonds's participatory research into the health visiting service of a south Wales community trust confirms the enduring nature of these tensions at the very end of the twentieth century. Writing in chapter 9, she explains that the origins of this occupation were in 'preventive' public health, and so its ethos was at odds with its organizational setting in 'curative' general practice, particularly where clinics were located in surgeries rather than in the community. Moreover, both public health and general practice were masculine realms in which scientific medical knowledge was regarded as the neutral foundation for the exercise of medical authority. Health visiting, conversely, was a feminized activity, the main object of which was to convey such expertise to the 'private sphere' of family child care and to police working-class mothers whose domestic skills were perceived as defective. For its practitioners, who often empathized with their clients, the contradictions between public obligation and private intuition were acute. Lifestyle advice, for example – a legacy of social medicine – was approached differentially, in recognition that telling women in deprived conditions not to smoke, what to eat or when to wean their babies was likely to be counterproductive. Strategies of negotiation and compromise were thus brokered in an effort not just to give meanings to professional encounters but also to construct a professional identity that bridged the troubled public/private divide.

The Welsh Dimension

Until the recent arrival of the National Assembly for Wales, medicine and health care in Wales operated within the British polity and the areas of policy reviewed in this volume shared a legislative framework with their English counterparts. But historians and social scientists no longer reduce nationhood to the state. As Geoffrey Cubitt has elaborated: 'nations are best regarded as imaginative constructs. They develop, no doubt, out of social and political experience, but they are the products of an imaginative ordering of that experience, not its revealed reality.'[34] Nineteenth- and twentieth-century Wales provided a particular social and political milieu for the transaction of medicine and health. The rapid industrialization of the south Wales Valleys, for instance, nurtured the kind of proletarian 'public sphere' that was able to support a network of medical aid societies which, whilst not unique to Wales, was more advanced than in other localities (chapter 5). Paradoxically, however, the 'imaginative ordering' of Welsh national identity was closely bound up with idealized pictures of rurality. Experiences of suicide in north Wales query this rosy image of social cohesion and moral probity (chapter 3), as does Russell Davies in his study of Carmarthenshire.[35] Yet the rural idyll remained durable, its assumed purity being captured as a metaphor for health. Therefore, it was deployed to represent the rehabilitation of industrially injured miners during the Second World War (chapter 7) and continues to be applied to the promotion of Welsh water, the nineteenth-century rhetoric of the upland reservoir now diverted to bottle sales (chapter 2). This emphasis on the rural in Welshness has not excluded the industrial areas. At the King Edward VII Hospital in Cardiff, for instance, there was anger during the First World War that government parsimony was denying Wales a medical school when Scotland, Ireland and England all had them (chapter 6). None the less, the rural/urban bifurcation has weakened the overall identity of a nation, much of which suffers the common economic and social inequalities of a marginal region situated on the periphery of Europe and hence disadvantaged in the global economy.

The secondary legislative powers that accompanied devolution are now allowing distinctively Welsh policies to flourish in response to these needs, even without the primary powers conferred in Scotland. However, it is important not to lose sight of the broader geographical perspective because inequalities in health and in medical care are an ongoing problem for the entire British Isles. Thus, in chapter 11 David Greaves posits that as the public health movement became medicalized in the third quarter of the nineteenth century, its mission was redefined to focus less on the health of the population and more on the provision of medical services. Suppressed during the inter-war years, the connection between health and social conditions was reconciled in the creation of the National Health Service which operated on the assumption that maximizing the care of individual patients would improve both the health of the population and inequalities in health. From the late 1960s, that optimism was challenged by studies which charted the re-emergence of inequality and culminated in the publication of the 1980 Black Report. But the newly elected Thatcher government, and successive Conservative administrations, chose to deny the evidence. Either they viewed health inequalities as an entirely private matter; or, if the input of other public services was acknowledged, there was a tendency to ignore the more deep-seated relationship with inequalities in wealth. Public responsibility was not reinstated with the election of a New Labour government in 1997. Despite commissioning the Acheson Report, which showed that health inequalities had widened, the strategy was to increase expenditure not through taxation but through economic growth. Therefore, policy embodied the contradiction that the public welfare and private market sectors were divisible. Wales is no exception to that dilemma.

Conclusion

In this introductory chapter, we have placed the study of medicine and health in Wales within the context of modernity, dating this historical era from the Enlightenment that took root in Britain from the seventeenth century and identifying its apotheosis in the welfare state of the 1940s and its belief in the feasibility of scientific socio-medical reform. Thirty years later post-war ideals were breaking down amidst economic decline, political disillusionment and a loss of confidence in the rational knowledge that had informed professional expertise. Whereas postmodernists revelled in the moral relativity of modernity's demise, Habermas sought salvage from the wreckage – hence his attraction for contemporary scholars. But though the concept of a bourgeois 'public sphere' rightly pinpointed the rising power of the state and its professionals, interaction between the agencies of central and local government was not disaggregated, and the 'private sphere' was a catch-all category accommodating the commercial and voluntary sectors as well as individuals, families and communities. Moreover, Habermas was elitist in overlooking the ability of the working class to construct their own version of the 'public sphere', gender-blind in ignoring how the two spheres differentially affected men and women, and insensitive to the imagined meanings of national identity. These myopias restrict the scope for the egalitarian, free and open communication to which Habermas himself attached so much significance as a mechanism for curtailing the bureaucratic penetration of the state and shaping personal identities. For all its shortcomings, however, the 'public sphere' shows that the historical and contemporary study of medicine and health in modern Wales cannot be reduced to a simple polarization between public service and private commodity.

Notes

[1] Porter, D. (1995), 'The mission of social history of medicine: an historical view', *Social History of Medicine*, 8, 345–59; Jordanova, L. (1995), 'The social construction of medical knowledge', *Social History of Medicine*, 8, 361–78.

[2] Williams, C. (1998), *Capitalism, Community and Conflict: The South Wales Coalfield 1898–1947* (Cardiff, University of Wales Press), pp. 1–8. See also Adamson, D. (1999), 'The intellectual and the national movement in Wales', in Fevre, R. and Thompson, A. (eds), *Nation, Identity and Social Theory: Perspectives from Wales* (Cardiff, University of Wales Press), pp. 61–5.

[3] Hopkin, D. (1987), 'Reflections of an editor, 1972–1987', *Llafur*, 4, 7.

[4] Dunthorne, H. (1991), *The Enlightenment* (London, Historical Association); Porter, R. (1990), *The Enlightenment* (Basingstoke, Macmillan); Wilson, A. M. (1983), 'The Enlightenment came first to England', in Baxter, S. B. (ed.), *England's*

Rise to Greatness 1660–1763 (Berkeley, University of California Press); Hankins, T. L. (1985), *Science and the Enlightenment* (Cambridge, Cambridge University Press); Henry, J. (1997), *The Scientific Revolution and the Origins of Modern Science* (Basingstoke, Macmillan).

[5] Rule, J. (1992), *The Vital Century: England's Developing Economy 1714–1815* (London, Longman); Wilson, C. (1984), *England's Apprenticeship 1603–1763* (London, Longman, 2nd edn); Barry, J. and Brooks, C. (eds) (1994), *The Middling Sort of People: Culture, Society and Politics in England 1550–1800* (Basingstoke, Macmillan).

[6] Borsay, P. (1989), *The English Urban Renaissance: Culture and Society in the Provincial Town 1660–1760* (Oxford, Clarendon Press); Langford, P. (1989), *A Polite and Commercial People: England 1727–1783* (Oxford, Clarendon Press); Owen, D. (1964), *English Philanthropy 1660–1960* (Cambridge, MA, Harvard University Press); Porter, R. (1989), 'The gift relation', in Granshaw, L. and Porter, R. (eds), *The Hospital in History* (London, Routledge); Woodward, J. (1974), *To Do the Sick No Harm: A Study of the British Voluntary Hospital System to 1875* (London, Routledge and Kegan Paul).

[7] Brewer, J. (1989), *The Sinews of Power: War, Money and the English State 1688–1783* (London, Unwin Hyman); Stone, L. (ed.) (1994), *An Imperial State at War: Britain from 1689 to 1815* (London, Routledge).

[8] Porter, D. (1999), *Health, Civilization and the State: A History of Public Health from Ancient to Modern Times* (London, Routledge); Wohl, A. S. (1983), *Endangered Lives: Public Health in Victorian Britain* (London, Methuen).

[9] Lawrence, C. (1994), *Medicine in the Making of Modern Britain* (London, Routledge); Loudon, I. (1986), *Medical Care and the General Practitioner 1750–1850* (Oxford, Clarendon Press); Cherry, S. (1996), *Medical Services and the Hospitals in Britain 1860–1939* (Cambridge, Cambridge University Press); Melling, J. and Forsythe, B. (eds) (1999), *Insanity, Institutions and Society 1800–1914: A Social History of Madness in Comparative Perspective* (London, Routledge); Bartlett, P. and Wright, D. (eds) (1999), *Outside the Walls of the Asylum: The History of Care in the Community 1750–2000* (London, Athlone Press).

[10] T. H. Marshall posited a move from civil rights in the eighteenth century to political rights in the nineteenth century and social rights in the twentieth century. For evaluation of this trajectory, see Marshall, T. H. and Bottomore, T. (1992), *Citizenship and Social Class* (London, Pluto Press); Bulmer, M. and Rees, A. M. (eds) (1996), *Citizenship Today: The Contemporary Relevance of T. H. Marshall* (London, UCL Press).

[11] Dintenfass, M. (1992), *The Decline of Industrial Britain 1870–1980* (London, Routledge).

[12] Ashford, D. E. (1986), *The Emergence of the Welfare States* (Oxford, Basil Blackwell).

[13] Barry, J. and Jones, C. (eds) (1991), *Medicine and Charity before the Welfare State* (London, Routledge).

[14] For fuller versions of the arguments rehearsed in this section, see Porter, D. (1993), 'John Ryle: doctor of revolution?', in Porter, D. and Porter, R. (eds), *Doctors, Politics and Society: Historical Essays* (Amsterdam, Rodopi), pp. 247–66; Porter, D. (1996), 'Social medicine and the new society: medicine and scientific humanism in mid-twentieth century Britain', *Journal of Historical Sociology*, 9, 168–87; Porter, D. (1997), 'The decline of social medicine in Britain in the 1950s', in Porter, D. (ed.), *Social Medicine and Medical Sociology in the Twentieth Century*

(Amsterdam, Rodopi), pp. 97–113; Porter, *Health, Civilization and the State*, pp. 281–313.

[15] Le Fanu, J. (1999), *The Rise and Fall of Modern Medicine* (London, Little, Brown), p. xix.

[16] Kumar, K. (1995), *From Post-industrial to Post-modern Society: New Theories of the Contemporary World* (Oxford, Blackwell); Lyon, D. (1994), *Postmodernity* (Buckingham, Open University Press); Leonard, P. (1997), *Postmodern Welfare: Reconstructing an Emancipatory Project* (London, Sage); O'Brien, M. and Penna, S. (1998), *Theorising Welfare: Enlightenment and Modern Society* (London, Sage), ch. 7; Pinch, S. (1997), *Worlds of Welfare: Understanding the Changing Geographies of Social Welfare Provision* (London, Routledge), ch. 6.

[17] Lyon, *Postmodernity*, p. 28.

[18] Hollinger, R. (1994), *Postmodernism and the Social Sciences: A Thematic Approach* (Thousand Oaks, CA, Sage), p. 155.

[19] Foucault, M. (1977), *Discipline and Punish: The Birth of the Prison* (Harmondsworth, Penguin), p. 27.

[20] Lyotard, F. (1989), 'Defining the postmodern', in Appignanesi, L. (ed.), *Postmodernism: ICA Documents* (London, Free Association Books), p. 9.

[21] Giddens, A. (1991), *Modernity and Self-Identity: Self and Society in the Late Modern Age* (Cambridge, Polity Press), p. 5. See also Leonard, *Postmodern Welfare*, pp. 32–60; Sarup, M. (1993), *An Introductory Guide to Post-structuralism and Postmodernism* (London, Harvester Wheatsheaf, 2nd edn), pp. 1–2.

[22] Hollinger, *Postmodernism and the Social Sciences*, p. 155.

[23] Habermas, J. (1989), *The Structural Transformation of the Public Sphere* (Cambridge, Polity Press). This synopsis of Habermas is much indebted to Steven Thompson.

[24] McCarthey, T. (1989), 'Introduction', ibid., p. xi.

[25] Habermas, J. (1996), *Between Facts and Norms: Contributions to a Discourse Theory of Law and Democracy* (Cambridge, Polity Press), p. 367.

[26] Habermas, *Structural Transformation*, pp. 27–31. See also Scrambler, G. (1998), 'Medical sociology and modernity: reflections on the public sphere and the roles of intellectuals and social critics', in Scrambler, G. and Higgs, P. (eds), *Modernity, Medicine and Health: Medical Sociology Towards 2000* (London, Routledge), pp. 46–64.

[27] Calhoun, C. (1992), 'Introduction: Habermas and the public sphere', in Calhoun, C. (ed.), *Habermas and the Public Sphere* (Cambridge, MA, MIT Press), pp. 1–2.

[28] Habermas, *Structural Transformation*, p. 142.

[29] McCarthey, 'Introduction', ibid., p. xii.

[30] Habermas, *Structural Transformation*, pp. 159–75.

[31] Habermas, *Between Facts and Norms*, p. 381.

[32] Kumar, *From Post-industrial to Post-modern Society*, pp. 174–5; Lyon, *Postmodernity*, p. 79.

[33] This paragraph is largely the work of Susan Pitt.

[34] Cubitt, G. (1998), 'Introduction', in Cubitt, G. (ed.), *Imagining Nations* (Manchester, Manchester University Press), p. 3.

[35] Davies, R. (1996), *Secret Sins: Sex, Violence and Society in Carmarthenshire 1870–1920* (Cardiff, University of Wales Press).

2

Public Utility or Private Enterprise? Water and Health in the Nineteenth and Twentieth Centuries

RICHARD COOPEY and OWEN ROBERTS

Introduction

It is ironic that the water industry was one of the last to be nationalized in the post-war period, and yet it is arguably the industry with the longest history of public ownership and collectivized control in Britain. The privatization of water in the 1980s sparked a great deal of new research on the history of the industry, and the ways in which complex ideas of ownership of this 'natural' resource have evolved over time.[1] This chapter will attempt to trace the municipalization movement during the nineteenth century. It will critically assess some traditional interpretations of the transfer of ownership of the waterworks of major towns during the second half of the nineteenth century, and of the rationale behind the large dam schemes which were constructed by great municipal corporations. In particular, the case will be made that the relationship between public health and the arguments for public ownership of water in the nineteenth century is not as clear and straightforward as it seems. The debate was profoundly affected by municipal power politics, rival ideas on political economy, and contested notions of territorial control. In addition, there was a great deal of disagreement over what constituted 'pure' or 'good' water. The scientific debate over pure water ranged from the evolving knowledge of water as a medium for the transmission of disease to the place of water (or indeed the best kind of water) in promoting health and physical development. Many of the debates of the time still influence the way we perceive water as a resource today. The chapter will focus on Welsh water but in doing so it is necessary to draw from the examples of the English municipalities which looked to the Welsh hills for their supply, and whose monumental feats of engineering have left such an indelible mark on the landscape.

The Municipal Imperative

During the first half of the nineteenth century, the period of the first real expansion in waterworks to cope with the rapid urbanization of the Industrial Revolution, private joint-stock companies were formed to supply the majority of towns in Britain. Only about ten of the 190 largest towns in England and Wales, Gloucester being one example, were supplied by municipally owned waterworks in 1846.[2] The situation in Scotland was somewhat different, an anomaly which was actually restored by the Conservative government in 1989, which allowed Scottish water to remain in public hands. The reasons for the private domination lay in the absence of local institutions with the necessary financial power and in the government's attitude at the time. According to Bob Millward, 'The evidence suggests that in the early nineteenth century the central government authorities, and Parliament in particular, regarded water supply as a normal commercial venture.'[3]

Competition between different water undertakings was encouraged, and several different companies were formed in some cities. In practice, however, it was soon discovered that competition was extremely wasteful, especially as the business of providing water proved to be less profitable than other types of investment owing to government restrictions on profit levels. Rather than having two companies laying mains in the same streets and trying to undercut each other's prices, amalgamations and agreements between companies rapidly became the norm.[4] In Cheshire, for instance, the Wirral and West Cheshire companies merged, and in both Liverpool and London the companies reached agreements over clearly defined areas of supply. Such deals were often accompanied by price-fixing arrangements.

Private water companies did effect a significant improvement in water supplies in many areas. They tended mainly to tap local sources. Towns which lay on porous rocks, such as Caerleon and Liverpool, often drew their supply from wells and boreholes; some companies abstracted directly from rivers, for instance those which served Wrexham and Chester; and some used existing lakes or constructed small reservoirs to impound springs or surface water, such as at Pontypool, Denbigh, and Mountain Ash.[5] The type and effectiveness of supply varied greatly from place to place, and in a number of towns the companies were heavily criticized.

The second half of the century saw a move away from private provision. From the 1840s onwards, an increasing number of towns sought to buy out the companies which supplied water in their area. Sometimes this was achieved quietly, while in some towns the companies strongly resisted being taken over. The peak of this municipalization boom occurred between 1861 and 1881, when the percentage of large towns with municipalized supplies rose from 40 to 80 per cent. According to John Hassan, 'By the eve of the First World War the municipalisation movement had transformed the water industry into one of the most collectivized sectors in the British economy.'[6]

The New Political Economy of Water

The public ownership of water, along with gas, became the bedrock of what was to become known as municipal socialism – a new political economy on a local scale. In order to effect this transition, a concerted ideological campaign needed to be waged. The traditional argument, and one which has persisted, was that this change in ownership was an essential part of the public health movement; part of the process of seeing water supply as a public good, and an answer to the obvious failings of the private water companies. It is often presented by historians as the answer to the basic conflict between the need of the water companies to make a profit and the need to have affordable good-quality water available for all.

Although the means by which disease was transmitted by water was not precisely understood until the development of bacteri-ology towards the end of the nineteenth century, it had long been realized that the consumption of polluted water could damage health. Epidemiological and statistical studies by Snow, Chadwick and others had linked contaminated water with outbreaks of diseases such as typhoid fever and cholera. Investment in water supplies was also needed if domestic cleanliness was to be improved, and if innovations such as the water closet and the self-flushing sewer were to be successful in improving public health in urban areas. A desire to improve both the quantity and quality of the domestic water supply thus became an important part of the mid-nineteenth century 'sanitary idea', and a vigorous debate was waged over how best to provide clean water for Britain's cities.[7]

The accusations levelled against the mid-nineteenth-century private water companies are well documented, and are frequently seen to revolve around public health issues. Firstly, it was alleged that the companies were reluctant to supply water to less lucrative customers, i.e. the poor. This did not simply mean preference for the middle over the working classes, but could mean preference for corporate users. For instance, there were persistent complaints that the Denbigh Water Company was always anxious to sell a supply to the LNWR railway company, while the least affluent residential areas of the borough often went without.[8] Complaints about high charges were also commonplace.

Another important criticism of many private water enterprises, for instance the Swansea Waterworks Company and the two Liverpool companies, was that the supply of water was insufficient. It was rare for companies to furnish a constant supply under pressure, even after the leading civil engineer, Thomas Hawksley, had shown in Nottingham that it could be done.[9] An inquiry held in the 1840s into the standard of supply in Liverpool heard evidence that the supply was only turned on for a couple of hours twice a day, and then at inconvenient times such as six in the morning. It seems that the deprived areas suffered most from this, and one Liverpool landlord testified: 'I have heard frequent and repeated complaints of the insufficient supply of water to my tenants, and on several occasions amounting to distress; so much so, that the tenants have had to go a begging in the neighbourhood.'[10] The inquiry found that 'it is a general complaint that the people have not got water to wash out the courts' in working-class areas of the city, a situation which had obvious public health implications.[11]

It is also alleged that private companies supplied water of poor quality and were reluctant to invest in new sources. There had been much investment by private companies during the early nineteenth century, mainly exploiting sources in the immediate vicinity of towns, but it seems to be the case that they were wary of building large-scale systems to exploit more distant reserves. Such a long-term investment was difficult for them for a number of reasons. The capital markets in London certainly provided the opportunity for raising large sums for the civil engineering and infrastructural development, as witnessed by successive booms in canal building and railways. Water companies, however, tended not to be very profitable, principally because the parliamentary Acts which incorporated them usually imposed limits on the prices they could charge. Parliament also limited the amount of money which the water companies could borrow.

Municipalization provided an alternative, and the impetus for the great water investment of the late nineteenth century. Economic historians such as Wilson have estimated that municipal debt almost equalled the national debt by 1914, a situation which was due in no small measure to investment in waterworks.[12] Municipal authorities' debt served as a low-risk, steady-return investment in the capital markets, and was thus able to attract substantial numbers of investors. Manchester and Liverpool were the first large cities to municipalize their water supplies in the late 1840s, and these two cities were to take the lead during the next fifty years in capitalizing on advances in engineering know-how to build huge upland schemes. These new schemes led to significant advances in dam technology, and the great elevation of the reservoirs enabled water to be brought to urban populations through pipe-aqueducts operating entirely by gravity and pressure, thus eliminating the need for pumping. Manchester built the pioneering Longdendale reservoirs, and then carried out a scheme at Thirlmere in the Lake District during the 1890s. Liverpool responded to its water needs by first building reservoirs at Rivington, in the Lancashire hills, and then the path-breaking Vyrnwy scheme in the headwaters of the Severn. This reservoir was the largest artificial lake in Europe at the time, took twelve years to build, and incorporated many novel engineering features.

Smaller towns and cities also saw municipalization as the solution. The municipalization of Swansea's private water company was completed in 1852, and was eventually followed by the construction of upland reservoirs at Lliw and Blaenant-Ddu.[13] Birkenhead Town Council also took responsibility for the water supply and, like its larger neighbour across the Mersey, looked to build a new gravitation scheme in Wales. The parliamentary Bill which authorized the construction of the Alwen reservoir was passed in 1907, although the scheme was not completed until the early 1920s. Some private companies did successfully resist the trend. For example, those in Luton and Newcastle successfully fended off attempts at take-over by the local authority, as did the Wrexham and East Denbighshire company, which remains independent to this day.[14] These companies were in the minority, however, as the municipalization of water gathered pace.

By the mid-nineteenth century, the need to move towards municipally owned waterworks was becoming the received view in government circles. A Royal Commission in 1845 was critical of private companies, and the 1866 Richmond Commission on the supply of London strongly advocated public ownership. An interesting example of this shift in official policy can be seen in 1851 in the case of Merthyr Tydfil. Merthyr had been without any form of properly organized general water supply until this time, and there existed a great debate over how best to meet the need of the growing town, which had been criticized in successive government reports as one of the filthiest in Britain. The great industrialist Crawshay and others wished to form – and control – a private company to supply the town with water, but the suggestion was received unfavourably by the government. The General Board of Health message to the Merthyr Tydfil Board of Health in November 1851 is indicative of the way in which the argument for public ownership was couched:

> When the supply of water is left to a trading company . . . the inhabitants are charged, not as they would be if they had merely to pay the cost of the service, but according to the extent of their necessities, and to the powers of exaction for supplying them . . . The abandonment of water supply to private companies involves the disregard of the public interest . . . wherever the promise of trading profit does not arise, or where the continuance of such profit may be threatened . . . the local board might find themselves entirely at the mercy of a water company with respect to the charges for water for uses which they may not now contemplate . . . These companies, having been formed by individuals

anxious for a profitable investment, dispose of it only to those persons who are willing to buy it at such rates, and on such conditions, as they are pleased to impose . . . Being a trading body, they naturally carry their pipes into those parts of the town where they can get the largest and best customers, and if the supply for the whole town is limited, the inhabitants of poorer districts where water is most required for the purposes of cleanliness and health, are quite neglected . . .[15]

Parliament also passed legislation which encouraged municipalization. The Public Health Act of 1848 allowed towns to set up local boards of health, and the 1858 Local Government Act made it easier for ownership of works to be transferred from private companies to public authorities. Later, the 1875 Public Health Act gave local authorities a statutory obligation to ensure that their areas were supplied with water of a reasonable quality.

Indeed, traditional interpretations of nineteenth-century public health improvements have focused on the efforts of central government and the 'great' public health reformers, such as Edwin Chadwick, pushing reluctant penny-pinching local authorities into taking action. As Ieuan Gwynedd Jones put it, central government agencies were '. . . slowly but surely breaking down the atrocious individualism of the localities and substituting mild forms of collectivism and state-direction for laissez-faire'.[16] This interpretation has generally been rejected by historians during the last twenty years. Hamlin in particular has highlighted the anomaly that local politicians are portrayed as lazy and reactionary by historians, while their achievements in the field of public health infrastructure were in many ways remarkable. He argues that 'what was recognized by officials of central government (and by recent historians) as resistance to progress was often bewilderment and frustration with technical and legal complexities and fear of taking a wrong step'.[17] It is now recognized by recent water historians, such as Bill Luckin and Mark Jenner, that the role of central government and its officials was permissive and enabling rather than proactive, and that much of the initiative came from the local authorities themselves. It is interesting that Chadwick scarcely merits a mention in Luckin's book on health and the environment in London.[18]

Most interpretations of the municipalization movement emphasize the ideological shift in the nineteenth century in the way people perceived the ownership of water. Water was to do with public health, and therefore could not be treated like a commercial business. Water was a good apart – not to be treated as any other economic commodity. This idea had great potency among many different interest groups, ranging from politicians to water professionals to public health reformers. The Liverpool Guardian Society, in presenting its evidence to the inquiry into the town's private companies, was of the view that 'the inhabitants ought not to be depending upon mere trading companies for a supply of this most necessary article of life. That . . . feeling, they venture to assert, is becoming general throughout the country.'[19] Joseph Parry, an Anglesey man who would later become water engineer of the Liverpool Corporation, wrote in 1878: 'The monopoly enjoyed by the water companies . . . is too often detrimental to consumers. Where the chief end of an undertaking is the profit of the shareholders, and there is no competition, the health, comfort, and security, of the public almost necessarily suffer.'[20] And perhaps the argument is most eloquently put by Joseph Chamberlain: 'It seems to me absolutely certain that . . . the means of life and death should not be left in the hands of a commercial company, but should be conducted by the representatives of the people.'[21]

Some historians have sought to present the transfer of ownership of water from private to public hands as a rather Whiggish story of progress and advance. It is asserted that municipalization was the obvious answer to a situation where private capital had failed to tackle the scale of the problem of water supply, and where public involvement was now seen as more appropriate than leaving everything to market forces. By mid-century there existed local government institutions with the necessary financial power, and an ethos of civic responsibility towards the health of the people. A change in ownership is presented as being a crucial prerequisite for the next stage of water provision, the construction of large reservoirs on distant hills to quench the thirst of the industrial cities.

Politics, Civic Pride and Monumental Engineering

Beneath this rhetoric about the people's health, however, there are many hidden agendas which profoundly affect the way that the municipalization movement in the nineteenth century should be addressed. Though, in John Hassan's view, 'the underlying reasons for the success of the municipalisation movement remain unclear',[22] Bill Luckin has shown that these debates over ownership and control are certainly related to wider factors in British power politics and 'larger political and ideological contexts', not just purity and health. Coopey has shown that, crucially, these local governments were also led by politicians who, in alliance with engineering firms, could see both the consolidation of financial power and the enhancement of their own civic prestige in, not just the control of water supplies, but also in the construction of monumental systems.[23] Central to these systems, in the case of major cities like Birmingham and Liverpool, was the acquisition and control of Welsh water.

Some of the hidden currents in the debate over water ownership and health can be best illustrated by citing the case of Birmingham, where water supply was municipalized in the 1870s under the influence of Joseph Chamberlain. Birmingham Corporation went on in the 1890s to build the Elan Valley reservoirs, which dwarfed all previous water schemes in Britain in terms of sheer scale and engineering audacity. The take-over of the Birmingham Water Company in the 1870s was more than merely a pragmatic attempt to improve the city's water supply. It also reflected the civic gospel of the age, the municipal pride and expansion with which Chamberlain's reign in Birmingham is synonymous. It is true that Chamberlain made emotive statements in favour of municipalization which attacked the company's record of supplying the poor, and that the goal of the municipalization policy was packaged as civic responsibility and altruism. However, it is clear that the political agenda of expanding the role of the corporation was also a major factor.

The Elan Valley scheme which emerged as a direct result of municipalization is in many ways a monument to civic pride. It was not the most obvious and practical solution to the city's future water needs, indeed it had to triumph over a range of local, regional and national opposition.[24] Big dam schemes such as these reflected municipal power and expectations – the system would provide tangible proof of Birmingham's status as a progressive and prosperous manufacturing city, and proof that municipal governance of the economy was modern and forward-looking. The scheme also reflected the lack of inhibition among Victorian civil engineers when it came to grandiose projects, and the alliance between Birmingham's radical politicians and elite engineers. It is also possible to argue that Birmingham Corporation regarded mid-Wales, like the colonies of the British Empire, as a source of valuable raw material to be used in the cause of progress – certainly to be colonized in advance of the ambitions of other municipalities, notably London, which had shown serious interest in Welsh watersheds from the 1860s onwards.[25]

Similar wider political dynamics shaped the municipalization bids and new water schemes of other towns and cities. By the late nineteenth century, municipalization and the construction of grand new gravitation supply schemes had become a trend, and the provision of water was developing into a contest or scramble for the best upland sources. According to the great Victorian engineer, Richard Hassard: 'In the manufacturing districts, every little bit of water-producing moor is strictly guarded, and each large town is jealous of its neighbours.'[26] Commemorative literature, produced to celebrate municipalization of waterworks or the construction of a new scheme, emphasized the benefits that would come from the council's great foresight. As a Liverpool publication modestly put it, 'No corporate body has been more fully alive to this great public duty than the Corporation of this City . . .'[27] Health continued to be in the forefront of publicity and served as a very potent justification for the large-scale systems. In subsequent years, for example, Liverpool councillors sought to justify the Vyrnwy scheme by pointing at comparative tables of death rates in various cities in Britain, and showing that after the scheme's completion, Liverpool had climbed steadily from the bottom of the list.[28] Issues of health and civic pride were thus inextricably linked.

The link between the construction of an elaborate public water system and ideas of civic pride and identity is clearly indicated by the case of Birkenhead. In 1906 the council voted to incorporate the town into Liverpool's water supply system. This decision was seen by many members of the public, and especially the press, as a surrender of municipal identity and independence. Despite the fact that the supply from Liverpool's Vyrnwy reservoir would be excellent, the debate was conducted in the emotive language of public health and of water as a public good rather than a com-modity. In the views of one whose letter was published in the

Liverpool Daily Post, water supply was far too important a responsibility to be bargained away for short-term financial savings. It was crucial for the health and well-being of the population, 'the lifeblood of the community'.[29] Birkenhead is an illuminating example. The way in which civic pride was manifested in the press and public opinion, and its effect on the town's authorities, clearly shows the potency and popularity of ideas of relating water, health and municipal pride. Water was clearly a symbol of civic prestige and independence.

In industrial towns, the self-interest of manufacturing representatives on the council could also influence policies such as municipalization and the construction of upland water schemes.[30] It was in the interests of manufacturers that the council could provide plenty of cheap, soft water for manufacturing, and water for firefighting. Commercial interests would also have more influence over the price of water than if they were supplied by a private company. Certainly, industrialists in towns such as Glasgow and Llanelli managed to secure favourable rates.[31] The evidence suggests that industrial interests were also influential on Warrington Council, who bought out the town's waterworks in 1890, and who unsuccessfully promoted a scheme to dam the Ceiriog Valley in 1923.[32] It may be significant that municipal investment in water supply, which benefited both health and industry, was usually given priority over types of public health investment which brought less tangible economic benefits, such as sewerage and the prevention of pollution. In some cases, municipalization also brought a profit for individual councillors who owned shares in waterworks.

One must also question the assumption that the corporations who ran municipal water undertakings saw their enterprise as being entirely in the public interest and no longer regarded water as a trading commodity. Cities certainly expected their waterworks to pay their own way, and although municipal waterworks were officially not allowed to make a profit, some towns did see ownership of efficient works as a way of reducing the rates, like any other municipal trading venture. Some towns, for instance Birkenhead and Warrington when they were formulating their respective Alwen and Ceiriog schemes, hoped to make money by selling surplus water to neighbouring authorities. It is true that Liverpool Corporation were reluctant to sell water in this way, but they certainly regarded their Vyrnwy water as a good investment and a valuable nest egg.[33] Birmingham's Welsh water scheme very rapidly made a 'profit' for the corporation, underwriting expenditures in other areas.[34]

Changing the Nature of Pure Water

There were, therefore, dynamics other than public health involved in the choices to control water resources and build big systems. But in order to buy out private companies or promote grand schemes, municipalities still needed to win the health argument, both before their own public and before Parliament. However, what exactly was meant by a healthy supply of water? Too often it is taken for granted that nineteenth-century politicians, public health reformers and scientific experts agreed on what constituted a proper wholesome supply. Historians of science and technology are now familiar with the ways in which scientific and technical understandings are shaped and conditioned by a range of social, cultural and political factors. The concept of pure water is a good example of this.

Christopher Hamlin in particular has raised awareness among historians of just how little consensus over the nature of pure water existed in the past.[35] Despite the mounting body of evidence that water was a direct agent for the spread of disease, the understanding of the exact nature of the disease-carrying agent was very poor. Miasmatic ideas, and theories which asserted that bad water was a predisposing rather than a direct cause of ill health, became less popular, but the available evidence was still compatible with many theories. People spoke of 'germs' in water, but there was little agreement on what the term meant – poisons, organisms or a process of decay – and there was no consensus as to which types of water were the safest to drink. This led to differences of opinion over which of the possible water schemes available to any given town would have the most beneficial impact on health.

As has been stated, a key argument in favour of municipalization was that public corporations had the necessary financial power to construct large new reservoirs on distant catchment areas; in effect to import pure water from wild rural valleys into urban areas. The municipalities therefore needed to construct an argument which emphasized that such upland sources were the best possible source of drinking water – far better than the local well or river sources offered by most private companies. Others, notably the private companies themselves, sought to challenge such ideas and the scientific assumptions on which they were based.

A clear example of this, of which there are cases in many towns in Britain, is the comparison between water from deep wells and upland surface water. Both sides could draw on conflicting scientific evidence to try to prove that one or the other was the best water for drinking purposes. The advocates of well water were also supported by the evidence of sight and taste – well water usually appeared to be crystal clear, cold and fresh. Those who supported upland sources, therefore, tended to claim that well water could be polluted by sewage seeping down from the surface, and cited chemical evidence of the supposed impurities of underground supplies. The response of advocates of wells was often that upland water was often minerally deficient. Opponents of the Birmingham Elan Valley scheme declared:

> The supply from the deep wells . . . is absolutely free from any form of contamination; it is pure bright and sparkling, and is considered the finest water in the world for drinking purposes . . . (and) contains just the right proportion of carbonate of lime, &c., requisite for proper bone formation; whereas the Welsh water is so soft that the health of our population, particularly of the children of the poor, will inevitably be impaired.[36]

This view is illustrated by the cartoon 'Wells or Wales?' (Figure 2.1). Similar arguments can be seen in Liverpool, Glasgow and elsewhere.[37]

Some advocated a dual supply system, where industry would be supplied by soft mountain water and drinking water would come from subterranean sources. In other towns, arguments centred on such issues as whether water closets or dry systems were the best options, a debate which had obvious consequences for a town's water policy. Some doubted whether a constant pressurized water supply was really necessary, and argued that having water in the pipes for only a few hours was ample. W. T. Foulkes of Denbigh questioned whether a piped supply was needed at all: 'children had been carrying water for thirty or forty years from those wells, and the exercise both did them good and kept them out of mischief.'[38]

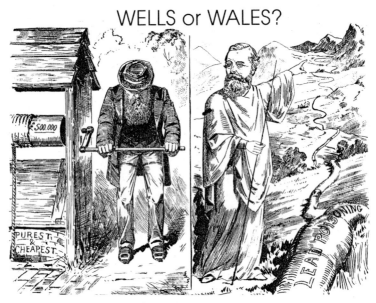

Figure 2.1 'Wells or Wales?' (*The Town Crier*, 1892)

A common debate was over how much water per day was needed for an average person to live healthily. In the case of Birkenhead, councillors were faced with having to evaluate the evidence of two experts who had very different attitudes on this question. George Deacon, the celebrated engineer who had been primarily responsible for the construction of Liverpool's waterworks at Lake Vyrnwy, asserted that forty-one gallons per head per day were needed, whereas the second authority that Birkenhead consulted, William Whitaker, used a far lower figure as the basis of his calculations of future water needs. This difference of opinion accounts for the fact that Whitaker came to the conclusion that the continued use of underground wells would be sufficient to ensure Birkenhead's future supply, whereas Deacon recommended immediate investment in a new reservoir in Wales.[39] Rival sides in the water policy debate, therefore, could both cite expert opinion to back up their case. Public authorities and water companies frequently employed rival water analysts to assess the quality of the drinking water supply – analysts who often not only disagreed about methodology but also about the very nature of water-transmitted disease. This was the situation in London, which up to

1904 was the scene of protracted battles between the water companies, who obtained water mainly from the Thames, and those in favour of municipalization and the development of upland sources. Edward Frankland, who, as Hamlin points out, had his own political agenda, was constantly critical of the standard of the companies' supply, which prompted the companies to retain rival analysts to defend their record.[40]

Central to this whole story, therefore, is the fact that the concept of 'purity' of water is negotiated throughout the nineteenth century. The people's health was, at least in part, a rhetorical device used to justify spending large sums of ratepayers' money on the municipalization of water companies, or on promoting large water schemes. The question of what constituted a healthy water supply was constantly under debate. Furthermore, the way ideas of purity were negotiated in the late nineteenth century has profoundly affected our ideas today on issues such as water purity and ownership of water resources. Today, Welsh water, indeed any highland water, is seen as pure and crystalline. Vince Gardiner has studied how contemporary makers of bottled water market their products: '[It] is never just water – it is more uplifting, it is veils of mist, it is dew dripping from trees . . .'[41] These are all images which can be readily identified in the settings of upland Welsh reservoirs such as Elan, Vyrnwy, and the Brecon Beacons. But the connection between mountain scenery and water purity has not always been obvious, and is to some extent a nineteenth-century construction. It has already been stated that water from deep boreholes was seen by some as the gold standard in the nineteenth century. People criticized Liverpool's Vyrnwy scheme and Glasgow's Loch Katrine scheme for supplying water which was peaty and brown, and Elan Valley water was said by some to be 'soft and insipid . . . surface storm water'.[42]

The construction of the idea that upland sources could provide water that was wholesome and good to drink is as great an achievement of the municipal water undertakings as the construction of the reservoirs and aqueducts. In preparing their case to counter the arguments of water companies and others, and in commemorative literature to celebrate the completion of great reservoirs, municipal corporations described upland water in the most favourable terms, and quoted from the most supportive of the scientists' conflicting reports. Language and imagery was used to support their case. Glasgow Corporation cultivated the link between Loch Katrine and Scott's epic *The Lady of the Lake*, and in celebratory literature to commemorate the opening of the Vyrnwy scheme, the water from the reservoir was not 'peaty brown', but 'pale sherry'.[43]

Until comparatively recently, the debates of the nineteenth century had also led to a public perception that water quality was best ensured by placing supply in public hands, and that water was not a resource to be traded like any other. This was the central justification for municipalization in the public pronouncements of local politicians in the nineteenth century, and the main grounds of opposition to the privatization of the 1980s. Even if one is sympathetic to such arguments, one must be aware that people's perceptions, of both water purity and the desirability of public ownership, are affected by a history of water supply in the nineteenth century which is overwhelmingly written by the victors – the municipal corporations. City authorities, during political debates over municipalization and afterwards, tended to overemphasize how bad the private companies were. Although the balance of the evidence is generally in favour of publicly owned works, one must not forget that many private companies provided a good supply. Bangor is one example, Newcastle and Gateshead another, and the Birmingham Water Company probably provided water which was excellent by any contemporary standards. A great many towns – especially smaller towns – were adequately supplied by private companies well into the twentieth century, for instance Bridgend, Pontypridd, Rhuthun and Rhyl.

Conclusion

It seems evident that municipalization was a successful solution to the need greatly to expand and improve water supplies in nineteenth-century Britain. Municipally controlled water undertakings certainly achieved a great deal, and the latest research does indicate that public investment in water supplies did contribute significantly to a decline in mortality from the 1870s onwards.[44] The history of how municipal corporations came to dominate water supply, however, is a complex one. Bob Millward, for example, has argued that there were many possible solutions, and that it is too simplistic to blame the private company structure for all the problems of water supply in this period.[45] Municipal ownership came about through a fusion of public health need, ideas of civic pride, politics and economic ideology on a local and national scale. Science and political economy merged, or were used to reinforce each other in debates which both attempted to reveal the nature of pure water and strove to set water apart from the laws of the market. The triumph of certain ideas of health and water purity went hand in hand with the management of local and national opinion in favour of the primacy of the public over the private – the dominant notion that water supply should be managed by the public sector. The water resources of Wales were appropriated as part of this process. As municipal triumphed over private, so scale triumphed over local. With municipalization came both the resources and ambitions which underpinned the monumental schemes which fulfilled the many aims of politicians and engineers, and which necessitated the control of distant, upland water resources. The ideas of the nineteenth century, and the way they were negotiated during debates over municipalization, still profoundly affect preconceptions about water and purity to this day.

Notes

[1] For instance, Millward, R. (1989), 'Privatisation in historical perspective: the UK water industry', in Cobham, D., Harrington, R. and Zis, G. (eds), *Money, Trade and Payments: Essays in Honour of D. J. Coppock* (Manchester, Manchester University Press), pp. 188–209.

[2] Hassan, J. A. (1985), 'The growth and impact of the British water industry in the nineteenth century', *Economic History Review*, 38, 532–5.

[3] Millward, 'Privatisation', 195.

[4] Hassan, 'The growth and impact', 531–47.

[5] For a study of the nature of supply in various towns in 1881–2, see De Rance, C. E. (1882), *The Water Supply of England and Wales* (London, E. Stanford).

[6] Hassan, 'The growth and impact', 535.

[7] Hamlin, C. S. (1998), *Public Health and Social Justice in the Age of Chadwick: Britain, 1800–1854* (Cambridge, Cambridge University Press); Hassan, J. A. (1998), *A History of Water in Modern England and Wales* (Manchester, Manchester University Press); Porter, D. (1999), *Health, Civilization and the State: A History of Public Health from Ancient to Modern Times* (London, Routledge).

[8] Pritchard, J. W. (1997), 'Datblygiad y cyflenwad dwr ym mwrdeistref Dinbych', *Old Denbighshire*, 46, 75.

[9] Binnie, G. M. (1981), *Early Victorian Water Engineers* (London, Telford),

ch. 8. See also Deacon, G. F. (1874–5), 'On the systems of constant and intermittent water supply and the prevention of waste, with special reference to the restoration of constant service in Liverpool', *Minutes of the Proceedings of the Institution of Civil Engineers*, 42.

[10] *Report of Evidence on the Alleged Dearness and Insufficiency of the Supply of Water in Liverpool: Evidence taken before a Special Committee of the Highway Board*, pp. 25–7; bound in *Liverpool Water Supply Pamphlets* (Liverpool Record Office), vol. 1.

[11] Ibid.

[12] Wilson, J. F. (1997), 'The finance of municipal capital expenditure in England and Wales, 1870–1914', *Financial History Review*, 4.

[13] Binnie, 'Sir Robert Rawlinson (1810–98) and the Swansea Corporation Waterworks', ch. 10 in *Early Victorian Water Engineers*.

[14] Bunker, S. (1999), *Strawopolis: Luton Transformed, 1840–1876* (Bedford, Bedfordshire Historical Record Society), pp. 108–9; Rennison, R. W. (1979), *Water to Tyneside: A History of the Newcastle and Gateshead Water Company* (Newcastle, Newcastle and Gateshead Water Company), *passim*; Wrexham and East Denbighshire Water Company papers, Denbighshire Record Office MSS, DD/DM/212.

[15] Grant, R. K. J. (1988–9), 'Merthyr Tydfil in the mid-nineteenth century: the struggle for public health', *Welsh History Review*, 14, 574–87.

[16] Jones, I. G. (1976), 'Merthyr Tydfil: the politics of survival', *Llafur*, 2, 19.

[17] Hamlin, C. S. (1988), 'Muddling in Bumbledom: on the enormity of large sanitary improvements in four British towns, 1855–85', *Victorian Studies*, 32, 60.

[18] Luckin, B. (1986), *Pollution and Control: A Social History of the Thames in the Nineteenth Century* (Bristol, Adam Hilger).

[19] *Report of Evidence on the Alleged Dearness and Insufficiency of the Supply of Water in Liverpool*, p. 2.

[20] *Papers of the National Water Supply Congress, 21–22 May 1878* (London, Council of the Society of Arts), p. 24.

[21] Quoted in Bunce, J. T. (1878), *History of the Corporation of Birmingham* (Birmingham), 409.

[22] Hassan, 'The growth and impact', 537.

[23] Coopey, R. (2000), 'Politics, imperialism and engineering: the construction of the Birmingham Welsh water system, 1861–1952', in *Water in the Celtic World: Managing Resources for the 21st Century. 2nd Inter-Celtic Colloquium, Proceedings* (British Hydrological Society Occasional Paper no. 11), pp. 375–8.

[24] Coopey, R. and Roberts, O. (1999), 'Engineering purity; the political–engineering nexus and the construction of the Birmingham Welsh water system, 1850–1950', unpublished paper, Society for the History of Technology, Annual Conference, Detroit.

[25] Ibid.

[26] *Papers of the National Water Supply Congress* (1878), p 17.

[27] Liverpool Corporation (1892), *Souvenir of the Opening of the Vyrnwy Works* (Liverpool), p. 2.

[28] *Liverpool Daily Post*, 20 July 1906, 5.

[29] *Liverpool Daily Post*, 19 September 1906, 10. See also the editorial columns of the *Birkenhead Advertiser* and the *Birkenhead News*, 25 August 1906, for evidence of opposition to the agreement with Liverpool.

[30] Hassan, 'The growth and impact', 537–44.

[31] Ibid., 542.

[32] For evidence of the strength of manufacturers' organizations on Warrington Council and their role in promoting the Ceiriog scheme see *Warrington Guardian*, 27 January 1923, 9–10.

[33] *Liverpool Daily Post*, 10 October 1906, 13.

[34] Coopey and Roberts, 'Engineering purity'.

[35] Hamlin, C. S. (1990), *A Science of Impurity: Water Analysis in Nineteenth-Century Britain* (Bristol, Adam Hilger).

[36] Birmingham Double Water Service Committee (1892), 'Why the Welsh water scheme is not the one for the city of Birmingham', 25.

[37] See, for instance, a report of a Liverpool Council debate, *Liverpool Mercury*, 14 August 1878.

[38] Pritchard, 'Datblygiad', 82. Joseph Parry has asserted: 'The idea of keeping the pipes constantly charged with water under pressure was very slow in its growth and met with much opposition'; notes for a lecture on 'Some problems of water supply affecting builders and plumbers', Parry Papers, University of Wales Bangor MSS, 20728.

[39] County-Borough of Birkenhead (1906), *Report of the Gas and Water Committee, Embodying the Report of the Special Sub-Committee on Water Supply*.

[40] Hamlin, *A Science of Impurity*.

[41] Gardiner, V. (1995), 'Water, water, everywhere' (London, Roehampton Institute), 14.

[42] Birmingham Double Water Service Committee, 'The Welsh water scheme'.

[43] Cox, A. (1892), 'History of the new Liverpool water supply', *Graphic*, 16 July 1892; Maver, I. (2000), *Glasgow* (Edinburgh, Edinburgh University Press), 91–2.

[44] Bell, F. and Millward, R. (1998), 'Public health expenditures and mortality in England and Wales, 1870–1914', *Continuity and Change*, 13, 221–49.

[45] Millward, 'Privatisation'.

3

From Private Grief to Public Testimony: Suicides in Wales, 1832–1914

PAMELA MICHAEL

Introduction

Suicide can represent both an intensely private deed, and a public statement. It is an individual act which has repercussions for family, neighbourhood and community, and so takes its place in the 'social' world. The fact that suicides show a distinct social pattern and that rates of suicide vary between different countries and societies has led sociologists to analyse the configuration of suicide as a social phenomenon. Durkheim argued that the incidence of suicide was a significant social indicator that could accurately reflect the nature and structure of a society. Although this chapter will briefly address the question of comparative rates of suicide, the main focus will be upon its public representations. It will argue that in Wales a powerful negative image attached to suicide, determined both by ancient beliefs and by the exceptionally strong influence of religion on nineteenth-century Wales. This inhibited people's willingness to recognize suicide, probably leading to significant under-recording.[1] It also meant that suicide was greatly feared and this, it will be argued, influenced people's willingness to send relatives to the new publicly funded asylums. This study is based upon sources relating generally to north Wales and in particular makes use of annual reports and patient case files of the North Wales Lunatic Asylum at Denbigh.[2]

Suicide was a crime under English law and a person found guilty of self-killing, or *felo de se*, forfeited their property. Lands and property were confiscated by the state, and relatives left impoverished. The law was modified in 1823, but suicide remained a crime under the English statutes until 1961. Because of this legal status, the full details of a successful suicide had to be reported before an inquest and, in this arena, not only the means by which the act was accomplished but also the motivation were considered. The thoughts and feelings and actions of the individual were subjected to public scrutiny. The law was mediated and enforced by citizens who were called to sit upon the jury, which listened to all of the personal and painful evidence before arriving at a verdict. Increasingly juries adopted the practice of regarding those who committed suicide as *non compos mentis* and therefore not responsible for their actions. As such, victims were deemed not to be guilty, since they were mentally incompetent, and property could therefore pass safely to the family. MacDonald has shown that by the eighteenth century juries had come 'to presume insanity instead of sanity', and Porter found that almost all suicides of the 'Georgian century' were routinely officially judged *non compos mentis*.[3] Verdicts of 'temporary insanity' did not mean that suicide was no longer feared, but they did suggest that in the public mind the cause was associated with mental illness.

MacDonald, in his comprehensive account of changing beliefs regarding suicide, focused on England, suggesting that 'folk beliefs about self-murder may have been distinctive in Wales and Scotland and stronger than those in England. They certainly', he asserts, 'endured longer.'[4] The evidence in this chapter supports MacDonald's position. The first half of the chapter explores how in Wales suicide was 'constructed' within the framework of various narrative accounts, especially those of oral recollection, popular ballads and newspaper stories. The second half of the chapter investigates how suicide attempts came to be redefined within an illness narrative, and were thereby represented as being subject to 'treatment'. It argues that the 'suicide rescue' was a powerful legitimating metaphor in the development of institutional care for the insane.

Wales Compared with England

Maurice Halbwachs mapped the suicide rates for England and Wales for the period from 1920 to 1926, and found that Wales had the fewest 'voluntary deaths'.[5] He suggested that the cause of the difference could be readily found by reference to a relief map. According to this ecological explanation the highlands of Wales, 'isolated, rugged and savage', were less conducive to suicide than the lowlands and plains of England.[6] Like his mentor Durkheim, he used the notion of advancing civilization and industrialization as an explanation for the increasing prevalence of suicide. He noted that Wales 'used to be more isolated than it is today', and that the difference between the suicide rates for England and Wales was narrowing. This demonstrated quite clearly, in his view, that as forces of modernization and industrialization advanced into Wales, the suicide rate rose accordingly.

Olive Anderson, in her book on suicide in England, similarly noted that, between 1850 and 1914, the suicide rate for Wales was considerably lower than that for England. She tentatively suggested that this was due to stronger social cohesion and more powerful cultural constraints in terms of family, kin, neighbourhood sanction and religion, and the absence of some of the social problems to which she attributes the higher rate in England.[7] During recent years historians have begun to challenge such assumptions of greater social cohesion in rural communities in Wales. Russell Davies has chronicled the extent of marital disharmony, interpersonal violence, poverty and neglect of children in south-west Wales during the late nineteenth and early twentieth centuries.[8] There was a serious disjuncture, he maintains, between the idealized image of rural Nonconformist Wales as 'a land of innocence and of absolutely pure and faultless morals', and the grim reality of life as recorded by court reports and newspapers of the time. It was a cruel and unjust society, he contends, in which unmarried mothers were frequently driven to commit suicide or infanticide because of their plight.[9] This we can recognize as the rural west Wales fictionalized by Caradoc Evans[10] rather than the sanitized rural idyll of some nineteenth-century Nonconformist writers, and latter-day promoters of heritage tourism.

This chapter will focus on evidence drawn from north Wales, and use the concept of the public/private dichotomy to explore some of the changes that occurred in the social meaning and significance of suicide during the modern period. Firstly, it will explore the shifting sites of discourse and changing representations of suicide.

Social Sanction against Suicide

Traditionally, both the body and the soul of those who committed suicide were cast out from society. The ceremony of burying the body at a crossroads with a stake driven through the heart 'had a religious and magical background of great antiquity', antedating Christianity.[11] This act of violence against the body of the deceased, and banishment from the community, was inspired by the belief that if a stake did not impale the body, the spirit of the deceased would return to haunt the neighbourhood. It was thus very much rooted in pre-Enlightenment beliefs concerning the relationship of the body and the soul.

This ancient practice seems to have continued longer in Wales than in most parts of England. Elias Owen suggests that up until the year 1823, when the law was changed, 'suicides were buried in cross-roads, at mid-night, without religious service, and the body was subjected to indignities'.[12] He had spoken to elderly residents of Denbighshire, one of whom remembered a crossroads burial at Eglwys Wen, Denbigh, and another from Gwyddelwern who could recall the case of a man who hanged himself being buried underneath the churchyard wall at night. As Owen observed, these 'sad occurrences made an indelible impression on the spectators'.[13]

Oral Traditions

It would seem that such burials lingered long in folk memory. Elizabeth Constable Ellis, daughter of the rector of Llanfairfechan, and a keen folklorist, provides one account. Although probably set down at the very end of the nineteenth century, many of her stories were collected from elderly inhabitants of the parish.[14] Tales of suicide, as well as those of other misfortunes, captured the imagination, and were repeated, becoming part of a rich oral heritage, fused with the local landscape. Typically the detailed stories describe the weather and time of day, and the prelude to the final act. Handed down through retelling, they formed a tradition pre-dating the lurid newspaper reportage of suicides. This is such a story.

> The weather was beautiful, ideal weather for ploughing, but the man at Ty Pitch had no horse to put in the plough. Suddenly an idea strikes him. 'I'll take the heifer, wife, and plough with her.'

'You will take the heifer? – my heifer?' She loved that heifer as a mother loves an only child. 'You will put her in the plough?'

'I will put her in the plough. It can do her no harm, and I must work.'

'If you put the heifer in the plough I'll hang myself', she said.

He knows she is half-crazed for the heifer, she always has been, but he goes out little dreaming the terrible earnestness of that threat of hers. He works with a will all morning till dinner time and then goes home. They buried her at the crossroads, but now the rectory hedge enshrines the forlorn grave, and the flowers of perhaps the loveliest garden in Wales scatter and burn their incense before it.[15]

As churchyard burials became the norm, conflicts over the interment of deceased relatives, whether unbaptized, Nonconformist or suicides, increased in intensity. Suicide cases, if accepted into the cemetery, were normally placed in unconsecrated ground on the north corner of the churchyard. Also, following a still older pagan custom, they were placed at right angles to the other graves, with their feet facing the east, ready to stand and face the Almighty as the sun rose on the final judgement day. This custom had extraordinary longevity. The writer can personally recall a case in north-west Wales within the past thirty years of a farmer, who was also the local postman, who hanged himself in his barn on Christmas Day. When the funeral party arrived at the cemetery, they discovered that the grave had been dug at right angles. There was consternation amongst the mourners, and close relatives refused to allow the burial to proceed. The body had to be returned to the undertakers until a fresh grave was dug for the following day.

In rural Wales folklore and traditional superstitions continued to influence the imagination late into the nineteenth century and even into the twentieth. In a land where people still believed in premonitions of death in the form of *canwyllau corff* (death candles), and in omens of death associated with the call of the owl, it was not unnatural to believe that the spirit of one who had committed suicide would return to haunt both family and neighbours.[16] Similar patterns of belief pertained in many rural societies and, as Minois observed, 'Everywhere, folklore gave a highly negative image of suicides.'[17]

Welsh Ballads

Y boreu dranoeth cafwyd hi
    Yn nyfroedd oer yr afon,
A darn o bapyr yn ei llaw,
    Ac arno yr ymadroddion:
'Gwnewch i mi fedd mewn unig fan
    Na chodwch faen na chyfnod,
I nodi'r fan lle gorwedd llwch,
    Yr ENETH GA'DD EI GWRTHOD'[18]

Curo'i dwylaw wrth ei gilydd,
A'r dŵr oedd dros ei dwyrudd lân,
Syrthio lawr dan waeddu Iesu,
O! maddeu 'meiau fawr a mân;
Hi ddywedodd cyn ymadael,
Cym'rwch rybudd gen'i gyd,
Dadau a mammau lle bo cariad,
Beidio'u rhwystro fyn'd ynghyd.[19]

Dygodd derfyn ar ei fywyd,
    Yn groes i lwybr yr addewid:
A'i law ei hun a wnaeth ysgariad,
    Rhwng ei anwyl gorff a'i enaid.[20]

Love and tragedy were favourite themes amongst nineteenth-century ballad singers. Broadsheets in both Welsh and English circulated widely, many describing the tragic stories of men and women who had brought their lives to an abrupt and violent end. Usually the ballads conveyed a highly moralistic message, in a still predominantly oral culture, underlining the dangers of deviant behaviour. This highly dramatic genre could be a powerful tool in reinforcing social norms and mores. 'The rejected maiden' was an immensely popular example.[21] It served as a warning to all young girls and women of the danger of seduction and subsequent rejection.

The period from the 1820s to the 1860s was the heyday of Welsh ballads. Singers would perform at local fairs and markets, and at traditional social gatherings such as *noson lawen*. Ben Bowen Thomas, in his book on the ballad as mirror of the age, maintained that these compositions, in the vernacular and quite unlike the high poetry written for eisteddfodau, were a natural and unpretentious expression of popular viewpoints. They took as their theme any incident, whether religious, political, social or personal, and spun a story around it in either an amusing or a serious vein. They dealt with matters as diverse as changes in transport, the building of bridges and railways, the growth of the slate industries, the impact of coal-mining, the introduction of the Poor Law, the 'Irish question' and many other topical issues and events. Taken all together, they reflect the width and breadth of the social experiences of the time.[22] Ballads played an important role in the development of a listening audience, and were a significant intermediary in the emergence of a nascent form of public opinion.

Without doubt the most popular were those which dealt with murders, and the ballads featuring male suicides tended to portray them in ways similar to those describing murders.[23] Indeed some of the suicides depicted were of men who had previously committed horrific murders. They picture them as aggressive, violent and selfish. The stories of female suicides, on the other hand, often focused on the wrongs which women had suffered, and portrayed them as victims of self-destruction. They reinforced the stereotypical view of women as dependent and vulnerable. The image of the poor woman, who is essentially honest and of good character, being driven to despair and destruction, is a recurrent one.

A suicide narrative could be used as a powerful device to locate the blame for this private act in a wider social context. In the case of the ballad of 'Mari Menmore' (whose subject died in 1839), the new Poor Law system was the ultimate villain of the story. The poor widow, left to fend for herself and her five young children after her husband was killed in a quarrying accident, was represented as the innocent victim. Unable to support herself and her dependent children, she was forced to enter the workhouse, where two of the children contracted a fever and died. She decided to leave, taking the three surviving children with her. Homeless and forced to roam from place to place begging for food, she finally fell to the temptation of stealing, in order to feed her starving children. Tormented by humiliation and overwhelmed with remorse, she drowned her children by tying large rocks to their feet and throwing them into the river; she then hanged herself.[24] This ballad, so full of pathos, was based on a widely reported story coming not from Wales but from Derbyshire. None the less it struck a chord in Wales, where people of the quarrying districts were only too aware of the ever-present risk of calamity, and the vulnerable position of the quarrymen's dependants. Opposition to the workhouse system was strong in Wales.[25] Sung in the Welsh language at fairs and other public gatherings, such a story could convey a moral message to ordinary people more powerfully than any political commentator ever could. Ballads often told how social change wrought havoc in the lives of individual human beings. In wedding the political and the social to the personal life story, it turned a private and personal tragedy into a public issue.

Newspaper Stories

As newspapers fought to increase their circulation during the nineteenth century, editors strove to appeal to a wider readership by providing lurid descriptions of murders, violent crimes and suicides. Thus, with the spread of literacy, the suicide story moved into a new genre. The detailed accounts of suicides produced in evidence at coroners' inquisitions provided a ready-made script for sensationalist journalism. In coroners' courts each morbid detail had to be officially recorded, and thereby became public property. The outwardly respectable appearances of families were scrutinized and contested in the public domain and debated over a wider geographical area now they were reported in the press. Never again would personal lives enjoy the relative privacy they had previously assumed.

Stories of murders and suicides gained increasing popularity in the 1830s and 1840s.[26] Over the next two decades newspapers replaced and superseded the travelling ballad singers, and the broadsheets. The growth of the press, so vital an element in the development of public opinion and of the public sphere, was inextricably linked with the changing discourse of suicide. MacDonald has claimed that the growth of the periodical press and the spread of literacy 'transformed the hermeneutics of suicide'.[27] It carried news of suicides to a wider audience, diminishing the role of oral tradition and communal rituals, and fostering instead a more secular and tolerant view of the act.

This process can be seen in Wales, and is well illustrated by the following account. In 1843 a north Wales newspaper carried the story of the suicide of a sixteen-year-old servant girl, Louisa Jones of Barmouth. On the day prior to her suicide she had been dismissed for 'bad conduct'. According to the newspaper, 'the vile practice of "bundling in bed" as it is termed seems to have been the ground of complaint.' This was a long-established courting custom in rural Wales, where the female servant class, who were expected to 'live in', were afforded the opportunity of courting during the winter evenings by receiving their suitors into the sleeping quarters. In cramped rooms the couple would lie on the bed, separated by a blanket wrapped around and between them. By the 1840s the practice was falling into disrepute, and was being castigated by both religious leaders and proponents of the morality associated with the new Poor Law, intent on reducing the rates of bastardy. On hearing of her disgrace, Louisa's father banished her from his house. It was established at the inquest that she had then visited the chemist in Dolgellau and purchased arsenic, saying that it was for use on the farm. Returning home whilst her father was out, she took tea with the rest of the children, carefully mixed the arsenic, and then ate it deliberately from a spoon. Despite the efforts of the local doctor to empty her stomach and counteract the effects of the poison, she died a few days later from inflammation and gangrene. The newspaper solemnly advised: 'Parents may carry resentment too far. We feel rather inclined to mourn the fate of this poor unfortunate than to expose and castigate her offence.' The jury returned a verdict of *felo de se*, and the 'poor creature was buried on the night of Monday, without service or ceremony'.[28]

Some attitudes to suicide remained hostile, reinforced in Wales by powerful religious sanctions. For a person to die by their own hand meant to lose the respect they may have earned during their lifetime. This is illustrated by the case of Charles Ashton, a village policeman in Merioneth. He was largely self-educated, but had developed broad intellectual interests. He contributed many learned and successful essays to eisteddfodic competitions, and became a noted bibliographer and literary historian. He retired from the police force in 1895 on pension, supplemented by grants from the Royal Bounty Fund and the Civil List. His entry in the *Dictionary of Welsh Biography* records that he 'died by his own hand at Dinas Mawddwy, 13 October, 1899'. Some biographers avoided mentioning this, stating merely: 'At the time of his death he was engaged upon a Welsh Bibliography of the nineteenth century.'[29]

At the time, the death was announced with suitable gravity in the local newspaper: 'Wales heard with painful surprise on Saturday of the death of Mr Charles Ashton of Dinas Mawddwy, known as the literary policeman, and the feeling was intensified by the news that death occurred by suicide.'[30] This was a measured, not a lurid account, and the article immediately set out to establish an explanatory framework. A correspondent stated: 'Mr Ashton burnt the midnight oil too freely with the result that his mind became affected, he being naturally of a nervous temperament.' It was explained that Ashton had spent much of the previous three months away from home, working at the British Museum and at the Cardiff Free Library, compiling his bibliographical work. He had returned from Cardiff the previous week, but planned to go there again the following Saturday, and so had visited the post office in Dinas Mawddwy, accompanied by his wife, to send some papers on ahead. His wife told the inquest that, on returning home,

> her husband had a foot bath, and afterwards cut his toe-nails with a razor that had been sharpened that day. When she returned to the kitchen to wipe the floor, her husband made a wild rush at her with the open razor in his hand, and in the struggle both fell on to the sofa. She got possession of the razor and ran screaming out of the house. Her husband told her not to shout but come into the house, and he would not do her any injury. He caught her and dragged her into the kitchen, where another desperate struggle occurred, but she again managed to escape by the back door, leaving her husband in the kitchen.

She then ran to the police station, and fainted immediately on arrival.

The policeman summoned the local doctor, and on going to the house they 'found Mr Ashton lying dead on the floor his head presenting a ghastly spectacle, and having the razor in his right hand'. The doctor reported on the state of the body. He had found Mr Ashton 'quite dead. He had severe cuts on the face, both hands much cut, and a terrible wound on the throat, extending from the muscles of the vertebrae and almost severing the head from the body.' The doctor explained to the coroner that he had known the deceased for many years, and that Mr Ashton's

> strange conduct at times had compelled him to advise Mrs Ashton about her husband's state of mind . . . He was very melancholy at times

and seemed to be nursing a wrong. He was also of a very excitable disposition. He formed the opinion that deceased committed that act in a fit of temporary insanity.

Mrs Ashton stated that her husband had been perfectly sober, not having touched any drink that day. Although he was depressed about his work, he nevertheless appeared to be in his usual senses, 'in fact, better than usual'. She revealed that he had assaulted her on a number of previous occasions, 'but only since his retirement from the police force. Previously to that he had treated her with the greatest kindness and consideration.' But at times, he had 'acted like a madman, threatening to take her life and to throw himself under a train'. The jury 'at once found a verdict of suicide whilst temporarily insane'. The body was interred in Mallwyd cemetery on Tuesday, the inscription on the coffin merely stating 'Charles Ashton, died October 13th, 1899, aged 51'.

At his death he did not enjoy the normal social ceremonies or public accolade of his achievements. Instead, the history of his morbid moods and his abusive behaviour towards his own wife was revealed. The jury was presented not only with a post mortem on the body, but also on the soul. What previously had been a private affair within the domestic sphere was now a matter of public knowledge, to be weighed and discussed in the wider social sphere. His private life was reconstructed as part of a wider social drama.[31]

It is not surprising, therefore, that families would become alarmed if a member displayed suicidal tendencies, and do their utmost to prevent a relative from committing this desperate act.

The Establishment of the Lunatic Asylum, and the Provision of a Safe Haven

The negative sanctions against suicide meant that families were particularly desirous of finding a 'solution' to the problem, and as the new system of public asylums was adopted, they looked to them to offer a 'cure' for suicidal relatives and to provide a means of prevention.

The establishment of public lunatic asylums was presented in the nineteenth century as an act of social amelioration, and of humanitarian concern. The Asylums Act of 1808 was a permissive act, facilitating the establishment of county asylums by decision of the county magistrates. This led to the first wave of asylum building, followed by a greater expansion when the 1845 Act made it obligatory for magistrates to make provision for their lunatic poor.[32] The North Wales Lunatic Asylum, although not completed until 1848, originated from the efforts of a committee of subscribers formed in 1842.[33] Dr Richard Lloyd Williams, of Denbigh, was the first secretary to the 'Subscribers' to the 'Hospital for the Insane'. He adhered to the philosophy of 'moral treatment', and became the first visiting physician when the asylum opened in 1848.[34] Prior to the opening of the Denbigh asylum, he and other progressively minded doctors from north Wales began sending patients to the Gloucester asylum, believing it to be at the forefront of the developments in humane treatment.[35] The medical superintendent at Gloucester, Samuel Hitch, in turn gave valuable support to the campaign to establish an asylum for lunatics in north Wales. Hitch explained how patients sent to Gloucester proved unamenable to the 'soothing influence' of words and advice at his asylum, since their first language was Welsh, and many of them could understand but little English. In consequence Hitch wrote a powerful letter to *The Times*, eloquently stating the need to establish an asylum for Welsh-speaking lunatics in north Wales.[36] It is a classic example of the utilization of the press to influence and mould public opinion in a way that would influence social action.[37] Indeed, it might also be claimed that, by recognizing the interests of Welsh-speakers, the moral crusaders behind the north Wales asylum were contributing to the discourse of nationalism that would soon emerge in the public sphere with greater force in the reaction to the Blue Books on Education in 1847. The institutionalization of a Welsh national identity was furthered by the success of campaigners, aided by Hitch, in bringing the Metropolitan Lunacy Commissioners on a visit to Wales in 1844 to investigate the 'special condition of the insane in Wales'.[38]

Some men, whose attempts at suicide attracted publicity, were sent from north Wales to the Gloucester asylum. They were members of the respectable lower middle class and their plight aroused considerable public sympathy.

Joseph Mellish was sent to Gloucester by Richard Lloyd Williams on 10th October 1842. An Inn-keeper and Tallowchandler from Denbigh,

Mellish was described as a person of 'regular habits'. About a fortnight previous to his committal he had suffered from 'excitement followed by depression'. Aged 58 he had suffered a double bereavement, losing his wife and a son. His four remaining children were alarmed by his suicidal propensities. He was sent to Gloucester, as a 'second class' patient in the hope that he could be cured.[39] At the end of the month one of his surviving sons wrote to Dr Hitch, asking him to reassure his father that both the business and all of the domestic requirements at home were being attended to. He expressed pleasure at his father's improvement and hope that 'through the Assistance of Almighty God and your valuable services . . he will be soon perfectly recovered'.[40]

The notion of the asylum as a haven, a caring environment where the patient would be protected from his or her most self-destructive tendencies, played an important legitimating function for the new asylum.

The Management of Suicide at the North Wales Lunatic Asylum, Denbigh

The Denbigh asylum, opened in 1848, rapidly established a good reputation both with the Commissioners in Lunacy, the public and many of its patients, under the dedicated supervision of its first resident medical officer, George Turner Jones, who remained in post until 1874. In the annual report for the following year his successor paid tribute to his work, noting that formerly there was a

> prejudice against Asylums: but the kind and efficient manner in which my predecessor managed this Institution for a lengthened period, dispelled that feeling, and relations at the present time do not make the same efforts as formerly to keep their friends at their homes. On the contrary [and he gives the illustration of a female patient] the reason for sending her, in the serious condition she was in, was, that her friends thought she would receive more unremitting Medical attendance here than they could procure for her at home.[41]

The protective and caring environment of the institution was often represented as the reason for transferring responsibility from the private to the public sphere. In the asylum the patient would receive twenty-four-hour professional care. The rule book of the Denbigh asylum stated unequivocally that the 'first duty' of the night attendant was: 'to ascertain the names of patients requiring particular attention, in the administering of medicine, or of comforts for the sick, and of those disposed to acts of suicide, and to visit all such patients every hour during the watch.'[42]

At the beginning and end of every meal staff had to count each item of cutlery, so as to ascertain that none were missing. Likewise, staff in the workrooms had to ensure that all implements were accounted for at the end of the day. The overall responsibility for all of the domestic equipment rested with the matron, who 'shall see that all knives, scissors, and sharp instruments, are kept by the attendants, and when not in use locked up'.[43] The asylum attendants bore the day-to-day responsibility for the prevention of suicide. One of their chief responsibilities was to 'ensure that security was maintained at all times to prevent both escapes and suicide attempts'.[44]

Patients considered at risk of committing suicide were kept under special surveillance at night, and visited every hour, along with those who were epileptic. In order to maintain surveillance over the staff responsible for ensuring this close and regular watch a system of 'tell-tale' clocks was introduced to monitor each visit (i.e. staff had to 'clock in' at regular intervals). The responsibilities associated with supervising suicidal patients contributed significantly to the development of systems of surveillance within the hospital. Not only were the patients monitored, but the staff too. A system of issuing 'caution cards' was introduced, adding an extra mechanism of formality to the transfer of responsibility, from one shift to the next. The caution card pertaining to an individual patient had to be passed from the attendant completing a shift, to the attendant taking over, who in turn had to sign that they had assumed responsibility for keeping that patient under close observation.

From the earliest days of the asylum, protection of suicidal patients against their own self-destructive tendencies was hailed as an important role for the institution. Freedom from suicide provided a benchmark on which to judge the efficiency of the asylum. At the end of the first nine years of operation, the medical officers congratulated themselves on the success of their institution in avoiding any death by suicide:

It is in no spirit of self-commendation, but with humble gratitude to the Giver of all good for His protecting care, that we remark the merciful exemption from suicide, with which this Asylum has been blessed – no case of self-destruction having occurred since its opening, and notwithstanding we have, in common with other Asylums, had many suicidal patients.[45]

Thus, during the early years of the institution, the virtues of asylum care were portrayed as having received a religious sanction, and as being endowed with the blessing of God. The medical officers went on to describe an incident when this 'happy record' was almost broken, emphasizing in their narrative how desperate the attempt was to commit the crime, and their skilful care in successfully thwarting the patient's attempts at self-harm. At this point a medical narrative began to supersede the moral and religious tone of the account:

An old man, upwards of 80, who had made several determined attempts upon his life before his admission, with the stratagem and cunning which marks the conduct of the suicidal, and which no vigilance can always prevent, contrived to secrete a knife about his person, and having entered a water-closet, he inflicted several most extensive wounds on his throat, one of which nearly severed the windpipe. Not satisfied with this, he cut himself in the bend of each arm, and on his legs. When found, he was lying in a pool of blood, pale, cold, and pulseless. He was speedily removed to a warm bed. Stimulants were judiciously administered, his wounds were dressed, and notwithstanding the extent of injury inflicted, and the great loss of blood, the old man recovered most miraculously, in the course of two or three weeks, and he has remained well ever since – but, alas! by no means cured of his suicidal propensity; and nothing but continued vigilance can avail to prevent him from repeating the rash act.[46]

This story was published in the annual report of the asylum. These institutional reports were circulated amongst magistrates and reported in the press and were used to influence and form public opinion, as well as being a marketing tool. They represented the public face of the asylum.

The protective and compassionate function of the asylum was given primacy of place in many forms of public declaration. Meeting at the asylum on 16 March 1860, the House Committee members deemed it their duty to record in their proceedings 'their warm approbation of the humane and energetic exertions of the medical superintendent in rescuing at great danger to himself a female patient who had attempted this day to commit suicide by throwing herself in the pond'.[47] This incident gave full drama-turgical expression to the notion of the suicide rescue. It presented the asylum and its staff as fulfilling a heroic role. The suicide rescue gave embodiment to the 'fundamental motif of an ethics of compassion'.[48] The asylum administrators cast their public reports in the language of moral philosophy.

The danger of drowning was ever present if patients wandered in the vicinity of the asylum. Most asylums were sited near to good water supplies, but this of course had its dangers. A favourite destination for suicidal patients at Denbigh was King's Weir, on the perimeter of the hospital grounds. Whenever a patient escaped detention, the large bell on top of the asylum would be rung, and the clanging chime would alert residents from the town, who would join the search. A reward was paid for the recapture of patients, and the annual reports regularly note the sums paid out for the 'capture' of patients. The arrival of staff and townspeople to search for and to retrieve the suicide victim made such an event a very public affair. It was also a point of interface between the asylum and the town of Denbigh, and ironically played an integrat-ive role, linking the asylum with the neighbouring community. It gave the local inhabitants a role in securing both the safety of the public, and the safety of the individual escapees. It served to unite care and compassion for the individual with care and concern for the public.

A public institution could offer a more effective means of preventing suicide and a more rational use of time and resources than the alternative of domestic care. Maintaining a watch over suicidal patients at home could be an awesome task, as illustrated by the case of Henry Evans, admitted to the asylum in 1881. A thirty-year-old agricultural labourer from Llanfaircwmwd in Anglesey, Evans was described as 'moral, sober and religious'. Following the death of his father and brother in a drowning accident, he became very low in spirits, and 'totally different in his habits'. He made several attempts upon his own life. For a full fortnight prior to his admission to the asylum, it was necessary to have three attendants guarding him constantly.[49] The time involved in protecting an individual at risk was onerous, and, in the context of nineteenth-century capitalist relations, increasingly costly. Details recorded in the case notes of the Denbigh asylum support Scull's contention that there is a link between the spread of a market economy and a growing imperative to place family members in institutional care.[50] It can be argued that industrial capital inevitably impacted on the domestic/familial sphere, diminishing the content and range of reciprocity, so that there was an economic imperative to transfer care to the public and institutional sphere.

In north Wales, the fear of suicide was a key determinant in the take-up of institutional care for the insane. As part of a wider research project, a sample of 10 per cent of the total patient admissions to the Denbigh hospital was entered on a database. The sample for the years 1875–1914 totalled 580 cases. Within this sample 127 cases were recorded as suicidal, either 'threatened' or 'attempted'. Hence, during these years, approximately 22 per cent of the patients admitted to the North Wales Lunatic Asylum had indicated suicidal intent, either by attempting or by threatening suicide. This is a higher proportion than has been recorded by other studies. The gender balance was roughly even, with sixty-five male, and sixty-two female patients registered as suicidal.

Contemporary analysts in the nineteenth century did not put such a high figure on the proportion of suicidal patients within the asylum. W. A. F. Browne commented: 'My own experience leads me to think that suicidal maniacs bear a proportion of about one-tenth to the other inmates of asylums. In a table of patients who have been under my care I find exactly this proportion.'[51] A study of a Parisian asylum found that an attempt or threat of suicide was noted in 12.5 per cent of cases.[52] However, the number of suicidal patients was not regularly accounted for in the annual reports of asylums. This may reflect the fact that admission registers do not always record the full extent of suicidal behaviour. Medical registers for the Lancaster asylum in 1842–3 indicated an average of 13.5 per cent of patients admitted exhibited suicidal behaviour.[53] Perhaps only a detailed analysis of the patient case notes (as used in this study) reveals the full extent of suicidal cases. If, on the other hand, the incidence was higher in Wales, then this might suggest that threatened suicide was a more important reason for committal in Wales than in England, and that this possibly reflected the greater fear of suicide amongst lay people. Also it might reflect a more powerful discourse linking suicide with sin. The asylum data would seem to be at odds with the evidence that accomplished suicide was less prevalent in Wales. Although not discussed here, an examination of coroners' records for Denbighshire has indicated that many deaths which might have been construed as suicides were not labelled as such. The fear of suicide may have led to the under-recording of actual suicides. It certainly motivated people to seek help in order to avoid suicides.

Many patients arriving at the Denbigh asylum during the late nineteenth century still attributed their suicidal impulses to diabolical influence. Samuel Wright was a 68-year-old blacksmith, who was suffering from the effects of old age, and grief at the death of his wife. The case notes recorded: 'He says hell is on his mind and the old Devil took hold of it. He attempted to commit suicide this week by cutting his throat. He said the old Devil persuaded him to do it. The Devil was strong and he was weak.'[54] In all 38 out of the 127 patients in the 10 per cent sample who had declared their intention to commit suicide evoked the Devil as a reason for their temptation. This supports MacDonald's observation that the belief that self-murder was inspired by Satan survived much later in rural districts of England and in the Celtic highlands of Wales and Scotland.[55]

Therefore whilst the asylum superintendent and nursing staff were situating the suicidal patient within an illness narrative, many of the patients themselves were continuing to manifest their suicidal urges by means of a religious discourse. Ancient fears and beliefs continued to influence the basic impulses of human behaviour, especially in rural Wales. Adherence to religious beliefs made people afraid of such diabolic temptations and compounded their fear of suicide. Moreover, patients themselves, terrified by the strength of their own impulses, would sometimes request admission to the asylum. In the case of a 61-year-old man from Abergeirw, it was stated on his medical certificate (part of the official documentation committing him to the asylum): 'he has been very depressed lately and he says if he is not taken to the Asylum he is afraid that he will do some injury to himself or to someone else. He is not safe to be at home.'[56] For suicidal patients the asylum was constructed as a refuge and a sanctuary.

Conclusion

This chapter has traced some changing popular views on suicide, and presented different narratives of suicide located in shifting sites of discourse. The sharpest discursive juncture seems to have occurred in the second half of the nineteenth century, with the development of the press, and the formation of 'public opinion' dominated by the middle classes. It ruthlessly sought out details of private tragedies which might be of public interest, and publicized them on an unprecedented scale. It drove friends and family to seek protection for those for whom they were concerned, within the mushrooming edifice of the asylum system. This profound change can be viewed as intimately associated with the emerging hegemony of the 'public sphere'. Instances of suicide were described, analysed and dissected, their social patterning was mapped and interpreted. Suicide attempts were increasingly located in a professional scientific discourse of medicine, sociology and psychology. Lay interpretations of meaning increasingly became subservient to professional explanations, both imitating their categorizations, and deferring to the professional for advice. It is argued therefore that the referral of suicide cases to the asylums played an important role in the professional colonization of life-world problems.[57]

Ironically the trend towards the 'medicalization of suicide' was the result, not of the claims of medical men, but of the decisions of lay members of coroners' inquisitions, who applied the appellation of 'whilst of unsound mind' to cases of suicide.[58] Rather than being seen as a wilful act, the action of suicide was designated a symptom of insanity. Significantly, nineteenth-century medicine offered no medical or pharmacological cures. Neither was there any consensus about its provenance. Esquirol, for instance, maintained that suicide was almost always a symptom of insanity, but that it was not a disease *per se*.[59] Routinely, in the case of suicides professional care simply offered a sound system of management and close surveillance. This emphasizes the key role of the asylum attendant in the multiplication of the asylum system. What previously would have been seen as a private and individual concern, became the province of an institutional regime. Suicide, the ultimate statement in terms of individual communicative action, could be deflected by correct management in a public asylum. The personal problems of the private individual who contemplated suicide could be silenced and contained within the bureaucratic framework of this new medical arena. The growth of the public asylum may be construed as a modern attempt to remedy life-world problems through system means.

From the perspective of concern over the suicidal patient, the growth of asylum provision during the nineteenth century may be placed in the context of the development of state welfare provision. It can thereby be interpreted as integral to the emergent framework of solidaristic provision. For Habermas suicide epitomized the dilemma of achieving 'the twofold objective of defending the integrity of the individual and of preserving the vital fabric of ties of mutual recognition through which individuals *reciprocally* stabilize their fragile identities'. The duality of concern of moral philosophy, of justice on the one hand (the subjective freedom of inalienable individuality) and of solidarity on the other (the principle of beneficence, of sympathy and compassion), could be explored through the example of suicide. Whilst

> this final, desperate act reflects the imperious self-determination of the lone individual, the responsibility for suicide can never be attributed to the individual alone. This seemingly loneliest of deeds actually enacts a fate for which others collectively must take some of the blame, the fate of ostracism from an intersubjectively shared lifeworld.[60]

In Habermas's view the principles of justice and solidarity 'have one and the same root: the specific vulnerability of the human species, which individuates itself through sociation. Morality thus cannot protect the one without the other.'[61] Habermas thereby recognizes the moral complexities raised by the issue of suicide, and addresses the question of the social relationship between the individual and the collective.

By the late twentieth century some of the stigma attached to suicide had begun to retreat. Headlines could proclaim the public confession of a popular Welsh singing star: 'I've thought about suicide' – 'Singing legend Tom Jones has revealed he once considered throwing himself under a train after failing to hit the big time early in his career.'[62] Public concern, and a growing sense of public responsibility over suicide patterning, again emphasized differential rates of suicide. The increasing incidence of suicide in rural Wales, highlighted by the figures for Powys, which showed the highest suicide rate for Wales in 1996–7, focused attention immediately on the social and economic crisis in rural Wales.[63] Social isolation, poor public transport, lack of social amenities and loss of jobs, were identified as the main explanatory factors. Farmers were found to be twice as likely to commit suicide as the rest of the population. This occupational characteristic was linked to the farming crisis, the weakness in livestock markets and the effects of the BSE scare. But a report also noted that 'The stigma may discourage farmers from admitting psychiatric illness.'[64] Mental illness remains the main explanatory framework. Reduction of suicide rates in Wales is listed as one of the prime 'targets' set for the new public health policy objectives. The aim was to reduce Wales's suicide rate by 15 per cent by 2002. The emphasis is now on preventive measures. Yet these measures are framed in terms of influencing individual behaviour, not of effecting wider social change.

Just as the asylum system was assessed on its ability to prevent suicide, so too the system of community care introduced in the late twentieth century was judged according to its record on suicide prevention. By the late 1980s and 1990s, 'reports of self-harm and suicide amongst those discharged from hospital suggested that community care was failing.'[65] Monitoring and surveillance were again introduced as a means of dealing with the problems, only this time outside the institution. Department of Health guidelines advised that an 'at risk' or supervision register be established in each community health area to monitor those regarded as being at risk of suicide or self-harm, or who were likely to commit a serious crime.[66] The aim had become to extend surveillance beyond the confines of the institution, and to regulate the everyday life of patients within 'the community'. To achieve this, the public domain must finally enter the private realm.

Notes

[1] An extensive analysis of coroners' records for north Wales, previously carried out by this writer, has shown that many deaths recorded as 'accidental' or as an 'act of God' could more plausibly have been interpreted as suicides.

[2] This article is based largely upon research carried out under a grant from the Wellcome Trust (grant no. 038862); see Michael, Pamela (2003), *Care and*

Treatment of the Mentally Ill in North Wales, 1800–2000 (Cardiff, University of Wales Press).

[3] MacDonald, Michael (1990), *Sleepless Souls: Suicide in Early Modern England* (Oxford, Clarendon Press), p. 142; MacDonald, Michael (1986), 'The secularization of suicide in England 1600–1800', *Past and Present*, 111, 50–100; Porter, Roy (1987), *Mind Forg'd Manacles: A History of Madness in England from the Restoration to the Regency* (Cambridge, MA, Harvard University Press), p. 234.

[4] MacDonald, *Sleepless Souls*.

[5] Halbwachs, Maurice (1978), *The Causes of Suicide*, translated by Harold Goldblatt (London, Routledge and Kegan Paul), 1978, p. 103.

[6] Ibid.

[7] Anderson, Olive (1987), *Suicide in Victorian and Edwardian England* (Oxford, Clarendon Press), pp. 98–101.

[8] Davies, Russell (1988), 'Voices from the void: social crisis, social problems and the individual in south-west Wales, c. 1876–1920', in Jenkins, G. H. and Smith, J. Beverley, *Politics and Society in Wales, 1840–1922* (Cardiff, University of Wales Press); Davies, Russell (1996), *Secret Sins: Sex, Violence and Society in Carmarthenshire, 1870–1920* (Cardiff, University of Wales Press).

[9] Davies, Russell (1983), ' "In a broken dream": some aspects of sexual behaviour and the dilemmas of the unmarried mother in south west Wales, 1887–1914', *Llafur*, III, 4, 24–33.

[10] Evans, Caradoc (1953), *My People: Stories of the Peasantry of West Wales* (London, Denis Dobson); Harris, John (ed.) (1985), *Fury Never Leaves Us: A Miscellany of Caradoc Evans* (Bridgend, Poetry Wales Press).

[11] Rosen, George (1971), 'History in the study of suicide', *Psychological Medicine* 1, 267–85, see 273. See also MacDonald, *Sleepless Souls* for a full discussion of changing beliefs and practices in England.

[12] Owen, Elias, *The Old Stone Crosses of the Vale of Clwyd* (London and Wrexham, Quaritch and Minshall), p. 74

[13] Ibid.

[14] Ellis, Elizabeth Constable (1988), *Fresh as Yesterday: Memories of Old Llanfairfechan* (Caernarfon, Llanfairfechan Historical Society, Cyhoeddiadau Mei). This book is an interesting example of early 'oral history'.

[15] Ibid., p. 28.

[16] This belief was still widely held in Anglesey during the last years of the nineteenth century; see Williams, E. A. (1927), *Hanes Mon yn y Bedwaredd Ganrif ar Bymtheg* (Llangefni, Cymdeithas Eisteddfod Gadeiriol, Môn); translated by Dr G. Wynne Griffiths (1988), as *The Day before Yesterday: Anglesey in the Nineteenth Century* (Beaumaris, G. W. Griffith). On Welsh folklore see Jones, T. Gwynn (1979), *Welsh Folklore and Folk Customs* (Cambridge, D. S. Brewer).

[17] Minois, Georges (1999), *History of Suicide: Voluntary Death in Western Culture*, translated by Lydia G. Cochrane (Baltimore and London, John Hopkins University Press).

[18] 'Yr Eneth Ga'dd ei Gwrthod', in *Cerddi Bangor*, UWB Welsh Library (Rare Books) (Bangor, Evan Williams), 190 (22), 'The rejected maiden'. English version:

> Next morning her cold corpse was found,
>   Floating upon the river,
>   Grasped in her fingers damp and cold,

They found a hasty letter: –
'Make me a grave in some lone spot
Where I in peace may rest in,
Raise there no stone to mark the grave
Of the REJECTED MAIDEN.'

[19] 'Cân Newydd yn rhoddi Hanes Galarus am ffyddlon garwriaeth Ioan Dafydd a Sarah Thomas', *Cerddi Bangor*, 22 (23). English translation: 'Beating her hands together, with tears flowing over her lovely cheeks, she fell down crying "Jesus, O! forgive my sins great and small"; before departing she said, "Take heed from me all of you, fathers and mothers where there is love, do not prevent them from coming together."'

[20] 'Cân Newydd – yn rhoddi hanes er galarus goffiadwriaeth am Owen Williams, yr hwn oedd ffarmwr a gyfaneddai yn Holborn, gerllaw Nefyn, yr hwn a ymgrogodd ar ddydd Sadwnr, Rhagfyr 24ain 1842', *Cerddi Bangor*, 326, 22 (80). English translation: 'He brought an end to his life, contrary to the promised path: it was with his own hand that he made the separation, between his dear body and his soul.'

[21] There were many variations on this theme. Other versions of 'Yr eneth ga'dd ei gwrthod' listed in the Thomas Richards collection *Cerddi Bangor* include 21 (113), 21 (114), 22 (46), 22 (47), 29 (32), Atod. 2 (20), Atod. 2 (95).

[22] Thomas, Ben Bowen (1958), *Drych y Baledwyr* (Gwasg Aberystwyth). 'Gallai'r mater neu'r digwyddiad fod y gylch crefydd, gwleidyddiaeth a bywyd cymdeithasol yn ei weddau digrif a difrifol ac o'u cymryd at ei gilydd felly, gall baledi'r ganrif ddiwethaf eu hadlewyrchu yr un gwastad o'i bywyd.'

[23] Ibid., p. 99.

[24] University of Wales Bangor, *Cerddi Bangor*, 22 (79): Williams, Richard (Dic Dywyll Bardd Gwagedd), 'Cân Newydd, yn Rhoddi hanes y modd y darfu Mari Menmore' (Merthyr, T. Price).

[25] Lewis, R. A. (1964), 'William Day and the Poor Law commissioners', *University of Birmingham Historical Journal*, 9, 178 and 180.

[26] Gates, Barbara (1988), *Victorian Suicide: Mad Crimes and Sad Histories* (Princeton, Princeton University Press). See pp. 38–9 for a discussion of the press coverage of the suicide of Margaret Mayes, who leapt to her death from London's Monument in September 1838. On the development of the newspaper industry in Wales, and the growing power of the press to influence public opinion generally, see Jones, Aled (1993), *Press, Politics and Society: A History of Journalism in Wales* (Cardiff, University of Wales Press), esp. ch. 4.

[27] MacDonald, *Sleepless Souls*, p. 301.

[28] *Carnarvon and Denbigh Herald*, 21 January 1843.

[29] Rowland, E. H. (Helen Elwy), (1907), *Biographical Dictionary of Eminent Welshmen* (published by the author). For an evaluation of the interesting career of Charles Ashton, as well as a brief account of the suicide, see the report in *Bygones*, 18 October 1899, 227–9.

[30] *Cambrian News*, Friday 20 October 1899.

[31] I was surprised recently to discover that this death is still the subject of public discussion in the area and that some local people maintain that Ashton did not commit suicide but was murdered by his wife. Oral tradition has extraordinary longevity in rural, Welsh-speaking areas of Wales.

[32] Jones, Kathleen (1972), *A History of the Mental Health Services* (London,

Routledge and Kegan Paul); Jones, Kathleen (1993), *Asylums and After: A Revised History of the Mental Health Services: From the Early Eighteenth Century to the 1990s* (London, Athlone Press); Smith, Leonard D. (1999), *'Cure, Comfort and Safe Custody': Public Lunatic Asylums in Early Nineteenth-Century England* (London, Leicester University Press).

[33] For a fuller account of the establishment of the hospital see Michael, Pamela and Hirst, David (1999), 'Establishing the "Rule of Kindness": the foundation of the North Wales Lunatic Asylum, Denbigh', in Melling, Joseph and Forsyth, Bill (eds), *Insanity, Institutions and Society, 1800–1914* (London, Routledge).

[34] Michael, *Care and Treatment of the Mentally Ill in North Wales.*

[35] For the Gloucester asylum, see Smith, L. B. (1996), ' "A worthy feeling gentleman": Samuel Hitch at Gloucester Asylum, 1828–1847', in Freeman, Hugh and Berrios, German E. (eds), *150 Years of British Psychiatry, 1841–1991*, vol. II: *The Aftermath* (London, Athlone).

[36] Samuel Hitch, letter to *The Times*, 1 October 1842.

[37] Habermas, Jürgen (1989), *The Structural Transformation of the Public Sphere* (Cambridge, Polity Press); also see Outhwaite, William (1994), *Habermas; A Critical Introduction* (Cambridge, Polity Press), pp. 7–13, 137–8.

[38] *Supplemental Report of the Metropolitan Commissioners in Lunacy relative to the General Condition of the Insane in Wales* (London, Bradbury and Evans, 1844).

[39] Gloucester Record Office, HO/22/70/Case Book, vol. 4, case no. 1377, date of committal 10 October 1842.

[40] Gloucestershire Record Office, D3848, collection of letters, 1828–44, sent to Samuel Hitch, bundle 7, letter from John Mellish, dated 31 October 1842.

[41] *Twenty-Seventh Annual Report of the North Wales Counties Lunatic Asylum, for the Year 1875*, Report of the medical superintendent, p. 12.

[42] Denbighshire Record Office, Ruthin, HD/1/70, Regulations and Orders for the Management and Conduct of the North Wales Counties Lunatic Asylum, Night attendants' duties, para. 2, p. 21.

[43] Ibid., p. 9.

[44] Nolan, Peter (1993), *A History of Mental Health Nursing* (London, Chapman and Hall), p. 57.

[45] *The Ninth Annual Report of the North Wales Counties Lunatic Asylum, Denbigh for the Year 1857* (Denbigh, Thomas Gee, 1858), Report of the medical superintendent, p. 9.

[46] Ibid.

[47] DRO HD/1/151, Minutes of House Committee, 16 March 1860, pp. 531–2.

[48] Habermas, Jürgen (1990), *Moral Consciousness and Communicative Action* (Cambridge, Polity Press), p. 201.

[49] Denbighshire Record Office, HD/1/362, admittance no. 3053, date of admission 22 January 1881.

[50] Scull, Andrew (1993), *The Most Solitary of Afflictions: Madness and Society in Britain, 1700–1900* (New Haven and London, Yale University Press).

[51] Scull, Andrew (1990), *The Asylum as Utopia: W. A. F. Browne and the Mid-Nineteenth Century Consolidation of Psychiatry* (London and New York, Routledge), p. 82.

[52] Prestwich, Patricia E. (1994), 'Family strategies and medical power: voluntary committal in a Parisian asylum, 1876–1914', *Journal of Social History*, 27, 806.

[53] Walton, J. K. (1985), 'Casting out and bringing back in Victorian England:

pauper lunatics, 1840–1870', in Bynum, W. T., Porter, Roy and Shepherd, M. (eds), *The Anatomy of Madness: Essays in the History of Psychiatry*, vol. 2 (London, Tavistock).

[54] Denbighshire Record Office, HD/1/362, admittance no. 3159, date of admission 31 August 1881

[55] MacDonald, *Sleepless Souls*, p. 351.

[56] Denbighshire Record Office, HD/1/382, admittance no. 8251, date of admission 1 June 1914.

[57] Habermas, Jürgen (1987), *The Theory of Communicative Action (Lifeworld and System: A Critique of Functionalist Reason)*, vol. 2 (Cambridge, Polity Press); Outhwaite, *Habermas*, ch. 6.

[58] MacDonald, Michael (1992), 'The medicalization of suicide in England: laymen, physicians and cultural change, 1500–1870', in *Framing Disease: Studies in Cultural History* (New Brunswick, NJ, Rutgers University Press); Porter, *Mind Forg'd Manacles*, p. 234, points out that almost all suicides of the 'Georgian century' were routinely officially judged *non compos mentis*.

[59] Rosen, George (1971), 'History in the study of suicide', *Psychological Medicine*, 1, 267–85.

[60] Habermas, *Moral Consciousness and Communicative Action*, p. 200.

[61] Ibid.

[62] *Daily Post*, 16 September 1999, 5.

[63] *Western Mail*, 17 November 1999.

[64] *Daily Post*, 14 May 1997.

[65] Payne, Sarah (1999), 'Outside the walls of the asylum? Psychiatric treatment in the 1980s and 1990s', in Bartlett, Peter and Wright, David, *Outside the Walls of the Asylum: The History of Care in the Community, 1750–2000* (London and New Brunswick, Athlone Press), p. 244.

[66] Ibid., p. 263.

4

The Early School Medical Service in Wales: Public Care or Private Responsibility?

DAVID HIRST

Introduction

The early legislation of the 1905 Liberal government has been considered to have challenged existing boundaries between the private world of the family and the public interest of the state. Three Acts, the 1906 Education (Provision of Meals) Act allowing for the provision of meals for necessitous schoolchildren, the 1907 Education (Administrative Provisions) Act, which contained clauses establishing a School Medical Service (SMS) on a national basis, and the 1908 Children's Act, all made inroads into the 'sanctity of the home'.[1] These Acts have been represented, in a somewhat Whiggish interpretation, as steps in the progress towards the post-war welfare state.[2] More recent interpretations of welfare history, however, have sought to emphasize the enduring nature of the 'mixed economy' of welfare. This has been expressed both in terms of a continuation of voluntary, private and informal welfare systems alongside, or in partnership with, government welfare provision;[3] and through emphasizing the differentiation between provision and funding of welfare in both a contemporary and a historical context.[4] In this context the Act of 1907 raises questions about the place of 'private' medical care, such as the voluntary hospital system, within a public medical service, and whether there should be state funding of treatment, or a mixed-economy model in which parents paid for the treatment of their children.

One issue immediately arising is the extent to which the new service was seen as necessary, or was motivated by concerns relevant to the Welsh context. Various explanations have been advanced for the emergence of the service. First, there was the impact of the Boer War and the consequent feeding of long-standing fears about the deterioration of the race, either with irreversible consequences, or at least with temporary but serious impact. Even though the Inter-departmental Committee on Physical Deterioration dismissed the wilder claims of the degenerationists, concern remained about the impact of poor social conditions in the conurbations.[5] Relatively few people in Wales, however, lived in areas which could be so described. A second foundation for the service, it has been suggested, might be in the drive for educational efficiency. A common, if not always overtly expressed, theme emerges from these initiatives; the idea that medical supervision and the imposition of standards made for a more efficient and effective system of education. The measures were introduced, not primarily for the benefit of individual scholars, but to promote what the pioneer Scottish proponent of school hygiene, Dr W. Leslie Mackenzie, called 'the increase of school efficiency'.[6] An emphasis on the connections between good health and good education can be found in other government inquiries of the period.[7] Finally, there was the spread of sanitary science, and the desire to control the school environment and prevent it from becoming a centre for the spread of infectious disease.[8]

Medical Inspection

The implementation of the 1907 Act engaged different groups of actors, parents, local education authorities (LEAs) and the state, in a series of contested areas: those of medical inspection, the provision of medical treatment, and the means of payment. A difficulty in attempting to look at the roles and attitudes of all the actors in the drama is that the place of the parents is obscured. Bernard Harris's history of the School Medical Service has been criticized for being over-reliant on official statistics and reports.[9] This is perhaps unfair – the School Medical Service was intentionally a vehicle for the production of such statistics, and was used as such for both reformist and conservative purposes during its existence.[10] However, the lack of specific documentation about the reaction of parents and guardians to the new state demands for access to their children to inspect and supervise their health makes it more difficult to assess parental attitudes. Some doctors were patronizing of working-class parents, some of whose less literate complaints provided good copy for the medical journals. Hence the medical readership were regaled with the letter from one mother saying: 'Dear Madam, I objects to my child being overorled by a doctor. I clears his blood vessels reglar with brimstone and treacle, and he don't want no more doctrine.'[11] None the less, from reading the reports of local school medical officers (SMOs) in Wales and elsewhere, parental concerns can sometimes be identified. According to the annual reports of the chief medical officer to the Board of Education, attendance by parents at inspections varied greatly, from over 90 per cent of parents to less than 13 per cent. Partly, this reflected differing age ranges and the relative efficiency of LEA arrangements, partly differing patterns, particularly in the continued employment of mothers. The Lancashire cotton towns had some of the lowest rates of school attendance. A very high attendance might indicate some degree of unease with the inspection process. More obvious indicators, however, were instances of refusal to allow children to be inspected. Though rare, there were specific triggers which seem to have induced outbreaks of refusal. Older girls were particularly prone to miss inspections, on grounds of 'decency'. Many LEAs employed women inspectors specifically to address this problem. Association with other less welcome government policies, such as vaccination or, during the First World War, conscription, also produced refusals.[12] The nature of the inspection was also an issue. Parents expected a thorough inspection, but they did not anticipate a clinical examination. Complete undressing of the children, or distressing procedures such as looking for adenoids by digital examination, produced parental protest. This was manifested when Dr George Carpenter, an unusual medical inspector in that he was a former hospital consultant, attempted these procedures during examination.[13]

Parents, moreover, disliked a private consultation becoming a public examination. In the early days of the School Medical Service, many people external to the actual examination, such as the head teacher, school governors, members of the school care committee and other waiting parents, were present at the inspection, which thus became a public spectacle. Few medical inspectors, moreover, had the sensitivity to the feelings of both child and parents displayed by the medical officer for West Ham, who commented:

> It is very evident that the children, in many cases, would feel ashamed to take off their boots in front of their school fellows. The privacy, here adopted, has regard to the possible sensitiveness of the child and avoids needless comment which might arise if it were carried out in front of others.[14]

Too drastic an approach also created problems: in Carmarthenshire, the financial and political repercussions of the school medical officer's action in excluding a number of allegedly verminous children from school prompted one councillor to complain that 'for hundreds of years the children had been taught in a dirty condition, and if they were going to take drastic measures to change the habits of the people they would only bring the education authority into disrepute'.[15] Previous attempts to exclude verminous children had been considered too drastic by members of the education committee, and in Carmarthenshire these children were allowed to remain in school, but separated.[16] This county provides an illustration of the difficulties, and sometimes lack of commitment by both officers and councillors, which could affect the School Medical Service in rural counties. The original scheme of inspection, using eleven part-time medical officers, led to statistical problems, as 'on account of the want of uniformity in drawing up the reports by the Medical Officers, it was found necessary to examine all the cards of the children who had been examined in the various schools'.[17] Problems continued after the council employed the county medical officer of health (MOH) as school medical officer, for his refusal to employ a subordinate to do the actual inspections led to many children being missed. Despite this, the councillors refused to take action, though after six years of dispute they were told that 'they had an incompetent MOH whom they ought to be ashamed to employ'.[18]

The Introduction of Medical Treatment

Bentley B. Gilbert has claimed the School Medical Service was not intended to provide treatment. Subsequent research by Hirst and Daglish has suggested the intention was always to provide treatment; the questions were how and on what financial basis.[19] Nevertheless, the encroachment on private family responsibilities weighed heavily at the Board of Education. The various drafts of Circular 576, the first guidance issued by the board, now preserved in the Public Record Office suggest a rather conservative approach to the issue of treatment on the part of George Newman, the newly appointed chief medical officer. Indeed, parts of the final preliminary draft resemble a Charity Organisation Society tract:

> The Board is of [the] opinion that speaking generally Local Education Authorities should not undertake direct medical treatment. There can be no doubt that a system of medical treatment, or as it would soon become, medical relief administered by the Education Committee might tend to pauperise the patient. And there are other objections. If children were to be treated as well as examined, the cost of medical inspection would be very seriously increased; and secondly, such action would almost inevitably lead to complaints from private medical practitioners.[20]

The draft went on to recommend the continued use of 'the existing agencies of the medical profession for the treatment of the defects revealed by inspection'. This would mean 'both treatment by private medical practitioners, [and] . . . dispensaries and hospitals'.[21]

Newman's draft therefore envisaged a severe restriction on the direct provision of treatment by the LEA. But before Circular 576 was published the draft was sent to Robert Morant, the permanent secretary, who then went through it 'line by line' with Reginald McKenna, the president of the board. Although most of the draft was approved, McKenna insisted the board

> put more peremptorily the duty to treat the minor ailments, e.g. ringworm, dirty heads, etc., without delay, as being a course obviously desired by the country generally; and (b) to speak of other and more comprehensive treatment as a matter for which proposals will be submitted to us by Local Authorities later on.[22]

The final version of Circular 576 gave a more positive view of local authority action, although assuming direct action would be delayed in all but the field of minor ailments

> 14 . . . The subject of specific medical treatment is, however, one which will require subsequent consideration in the light of the findings of medical inspection and the collateral issues raised thereby, and it is clear that, speaking generally . . . Local Education Authorities will be unable to formulate . . . any comprehensive scheme for the furtherance of this object until they have considered the results of their medical inspection in various directions.
>
> 15 In the meantime, the authorities should take measures without delay, for dealing through such agencies as are conveniently available, with what are commonly, though in a sense erroneously, regarded as minor ailments.[23]

In practice the board did not receive many applications for permission to begin treatment in the first months of the School Medical Service. Many LEAs had yet to begin inspection, and others were reluctant to do more in the absence of grant aid. Newman developed his ideas in Circular 596, published in August 1908.[24] The preliminary discussions again suggest a conservative approach. He argued that the

> Primary duty of the state is to point out defects and disease and . . . to leave treatment as far as possible to the ordinary channels and therapeutics and particularly to those channels which increase rather than decrease the sense of responsibility in the parents and guardians of the children.[25]

Any work done should have an 'educational character', limiting the School Medical Service to problems with a direct bearing on school achievement. Within these boundaries, direct intervention by the local authority should be restricted, and allowed only in cases where it could not otherwise be provided effectively and efficiently. In Newman's view, this restricted the possibilities to eyesight testing, verminous conditions, skin diseases and minor ailments. Tonsils and adenoids, and dentistry, were marginal cases.[26] In the absence of LEA provision, treatment opportunities for many elementary schoolchildren were limited. Only the better-off parents were likely to pay for a family doctor.[27]

In many cases the recommended treatment made the GP an impracticable option. For discharging ears (otitis media) it was recommended that the ears be syringed up to three times daily, while some eye and skin infections needed similar regular or prolonged medical care. Other conditions, such as badly decayed teeth, were not normally dealt with by general practitioners.[28] Some school medical officers, in Wales and elsewhere, were deaf to the real need for medical care. The SMO for Denbighshire reported:

> the great majority, if not all, of the children in the county can easily obtain treatment from private practitioners. In the industrial districts of East Denbighshire they are attended by the colliery surgeons. There are also two excellent General Hospitals, one in the Eastern and one in the Western portion of the county where treatment of a specialist character can be carried out. It is felt, however that if possible it would be wise not to trespass on the sphere of the family medical practitioners.[29]

Parents usually turned to the outpatient departments of the voluntary hospitals. Newman noted the 'greatly increased' use of hospitals and other medical charities by schoolchildren and their parents.[30] Some voluntary hospitals reacted by not treating schoolchildren at all.[31] Other sections of the medical community were also opposed to the use of the outpatient departments. GPs believed that the increasing use of these facilities occurred at the expense of the practice and income of the family doctor.[32]

The increasing reluctance of the voluntary hospitals to treat schoolchildren was not only due to the obvious pressures on staff. To some, it was an abuse of their charitable role of treating the 'necessitous poor'.[33] For hospitals, the arrival of the schoolchildren after medical inspection was a perversion of the role of the outpatient departments to provide a pool of patients with 'interesting' diseases which could be selected and referred on for further study. Now, after the 1907 Act, there was also the question of whether the local authority itself should be undertaking treatment.

Apart from the problems created for the hospitals, the use of outpatient departments also presented difficulties for parents. Getting treatment might entail a protracted preliminary search for a 'ticket' from a hospital subscriber, if the parent was not a member of the 'Hospital Saturday Fund' or a similar workplace-based subscription scheme. Unaccompanied children were not treated, so taking the child to hospital would lead to loss of earnings and travelling expenses, often repeatedly; even a prescription for spectacles needed at least two visits. The notoriously overcrowded waiting rooms of the outpatient departments meant that it was often a matter of chance whether a consultation was obtained, and parents were often disappointed. When a child was seen, examination was often cursory, and the prescriptions issued sometimes needlessly expensive, elaborate or inappropriate. Although these obstacles could be overcome by an agreement between the education authority and hospital, these arrangements tended to be made to suit the convenience of the hospital and its staff, not the child patients.

Many children could not use an outpatient department, for many areas were far away from the nearest voluntary hospital. For an Abertillery child to visit the outpatient department at the nearest voluntary hospital in Newport meant a seventeen-mile train journey.[34]

Existing avenues of treatment of schoolchildren therefore had two main defects. First, one or more of a number of barriers had to be surmounted. These might be financial, such as a requirement to pay fees, or prepayment of subscriptions; they might be the administrative deterrence symbolized by the regulations of the Poor Law,[35] or they might be other administrative, geographical or structural barriers, including the travelling distance to a treatment centre or the difficulties of obtaining a consultation in the crowded hospital outpatient department. Second, the existing institutions were unsuited to treat many of the most common conditions of schoolchildren. They needed continual attention or required simple but effective remedial action, rather than the sophisticated approach sometimes taken by the voluntary hospitals.

Medical inspection also reduced the income of the LEAs by identifying children suffering from infectious or contagious diseases who should not have been attending school. Exclusion of these children meant that the local authority lost education grant income. In the case of a disease like ringworm, exclusion could lead to the loss of a significant amount of grant. The usual treatment by ointments was unsatisfactory, resulting in persistence of the disease. In Shropshire, the school medical officer reported in 1915 that 'three children have been absent from school off and on for more than six years, five for five years, ten for four years, seventeen for three years, and thirty two for two years, on account of ringworm'.[36] The resulting loss of grant led to a suggestion that it would pay the authority to arrange for the treatment of affected children by X-rays, which could produce a cure within weeks.

Some local authorities resorted to coercive action to force parents to obtain treatment for their children, though this was usually confined to cases of vermin and, less frequently, ringworm. Action under the School Attendance Acts meant excluding children from school until they were sent back free from the affliction. Parents who failed to deal with the problem were then summonsed for failing to send their children to school.[37] In West Bromwich, the stipendiary magistrate declared it the 'mother's duty to take care of her children and keep them clean and free from vermin and the father's duty to see the mother did hers' before fining the fathers and sentencing the mothers to twenty-one days' hard labour.[38] The difficulty with such coercive measures was again their effect on the average attendance. This sometimes brought the school medical officer and the members and officers of the education committee into conflict, as in Carmarthenshire, noted above.

Mutuality and Charitable Provision

The need to provide treatment for schoolchildren after medical inspection following the establishment of the School Medical Service under the 1907 Education (Administrative Provisions) Act led to a debate on whether public or private provision was the best way forward. The debate was not only about the most effective way of providing treatment; different systems produced ideological and political dilemmas for some policy-makers. While the establishment of school clinics was supported by many on purely practical grounds as the best means of ensuring that schoolchildren were treated, the fact that clinics were both provided and funded by the LEAs led others to attack them as being characteristic of 'municipal socialism'.[39] Such considerations led the Moderate (Conservative) administration of the London County Council (LCC) to arrange treatment through the voluntary hospitals of the capital, rather than to develop the pioneering clinics operated within the LCC area by the socialist educational reformer

Margaret McMillan, and others.[40] For some, however, even an arrangement with the hospitals was fundamentally unsatisfactory, for while this might ensure that the treatment was provided by a voluntary body, it was still funded by the local authority. This outright rejection of state intervention led to interest in schemes which emphasized parental responsibility by being both provided and funded independently of the LEA through collective, providential planning. Enthusiastic supporters of such self-help schemes suggested that the remedy lay in the formation of Junior Provident Societies, with children paying between 2d and 6d a month for full benefit cover. In London, advocates of the insurance principle attempted to persuade the LCC to adopt this approach. In evidence to a subcommittee of the Education Committee looking at the best way to provide treatment for the schoolchildren of the capital their spokesman, T. Hancock Nunn, a leading member of the Charity Organisation Society, claimed that 50 per cent of the child population of Hampstead were Junior Foresters already, adding that 'neither Jews nor aliens were excluded' from membership.[41]

While the LCC rejected these proposals in favour of direct arrangements with the voluntary hospitals, in other areas more determined efforts were made to develop a providential system. In Derbyshire Dr Sydney Barwise, the county medical officer of health, was a strong supporter of the idea. Barwise was able to provide a justification. 'The provision of such a service as is required by a co-operative movement in which parents and their neighbours interested in the health of the children joined, is in accordance with the particular genius of the English people – it makes for independence and character.'[42] Similar sentiments were expressed by proponents of insurance-based systems elsewhere in the country. In Caernarfonshire the justification was the altruistic sense developed in the children: 'it is believed that [a Medical Relief Fund] will engender and develop in the minds and hearts of the children a desire to help each other. Children . . . will have the privilege of assisting in providing means to lessen suffering . . .'[43]

Despite the hopes of the promoters, setting up a mutual aid scheme for schoolchildren proved difficult. Under the provisions of the 1907 Act, all treatment schemes which had an element of LEA funding had to be approved by the Board of Education. The subsidy inherent in the Derbyshire scheme meant that it required the sanction of the board. The Derbyshire scheme was sanctioned, but when the Caernarfonshire County Council asked for approval of a similar scheme, to be called the Caernarfonshire Children's Medical Relief Fund, the board reappraised its policy. The fundamental problem was the medical club's need for an initial injection of funds from the education authority to pay for publicity and working capital, although the object was to establish a self-supporting scheme. The board's sanction was needed for this initial contribution, and this caused some discussion about the problems of principle involved. All ratepayers were being asked to contribute to a scheme from which only those children whose parents subscribed would eventually derive benefit. The Welsh Department of the board supported the proposal, but the eventual consensus view within the board was that it was unable to

> defend a scheme under which the local education authority would contribute towards the expenses of treating children whose parents could afford to pay something in advance towards the cost of such treatment while they would refuse to provide or contribute toward the cost of the residue of children whose parents were either unwilling or unable to pay the cost of treatment in advance.[44]

Once the principle of full funding by the contributors was abandoned, the ratepayers of the county were subsidizing individuals or schools contributing to the system, while declining to help those who did not contribute. The children of the poor would not only have lost access to medical care, they would have seen the children of those with the funds to contribute subsidized for so doing.

Despite the board's refusal to sanction the Caernarfonshire scheme, some attempt was made within the county to continue to collect subscriptions until 1914 at least. A subscription book for Bontnewydd school survives, and shows that even in 1911, the first year of the Caernarfonshire scheme and the one in which the highest percentage of children contributed, many subscribers paid only one subscription.[45] Even in this year, the uptake of the scheme varied considerably between schools, from almost 100 per cent payment of one subscription at least, to schools with virtually no subscribers.[46] The subcommittee resolved to give help from the fund only to subscribers,[47] but with treatment for many items increasingly available through the School Medical Service in Caernarfonshire, payments from the fund seem increasingly to have been used to pay for operations, X-ray treatment of ringworm, and the payment of expenses to parents accompanying their children to treatment.[48] Restriction of payments to a small number of expensive items would have further reduced the attraction of subscribing to many parents.

The refusal of the Board of Education to sanction schemes which would have excluded the children of the poor, or those who chose not to contribute, from benefit was a key administrative cause of the failure of mutual benefit schemes to develop in the School Medical Service. When grant aid for medical treatment under the School Medical Service became available, in the 1912–13 financial year, they were ineligible for support because they were contributory schemes.[49]

None the less, most contributory benefit schemes seem to have failed not because of administrative opposition, but because they could not attract the support of parents. This may have been a symptom of the general decline in allegiance to the friendly-society movement at this time, but it was also due to the inapplicability of aspects of the concept of mutuality to school health. As individual subscribers, parents wanted some benefit to accrue to their own children. Due to the medical inspection system, they were able to judge how far their children might need medical aid, and to that extent, the idea of guarding against unexpected eventualities embedded in the friendly-society system was absent. As mutual subscribers, however, parents were unwilling to see benefits go to the children of those who did not subscribe.

The proposals for provident provision for schoolchildren ultimately failed, but they shed light on the opposition which existed to the extension of state welfare provision even in those areas where, in the aftermath of the Boer War, there was the greatest consensus that something had to be done. They showed the survival of the values of the friendly societies even at a time when those values were under increasing strain. It is notable that the two areas discussed in this chapter contained large mining/quarrying communities where the friendly-society movement was strong.

Public Provision of Treatment for Schoolchildren

With neither the voluntary hospitals nor mutual benefit schemes providing a solution, publicly provided school clinics gradually grew in number, though, strictly interpreted, Circular 596 required authorities to explore alternatives before themselves providing clinics. The concept of a school clinic in England and Wales derived from two main sources, socialist idealism and the Prussian example. The former was present from the 1880s onwards in the policies of the various emergent labour and socialist organizations. These urged the provision of free school meals and medical treatment as part of a programme of 'state maintenance' for schoolchildren. In 1906, the Social Democratic Federation was repeating long-standing policies when it pledged

> to continue with redoubled vigour the agitation in favour of state maintenance for schoolchildren, and to urge on the Board of Education the necessity of such an extension of the physical side of education as shall place skilled medical advice within the reach of every child, and, by systematic medical inspection, secure records of the physical development of the children attending state supported schools.[50]

Margaret McMillan also persuaded Joseph Fels, the Naphtha Soap tycoon, to fund an experimental school clinic at Devons Road school, Bow. Although pioneering in its intentions, the small attendance at the clinic after its inauguration in 1908 threatened to portray it as a high-cost method of treatment, and so in March 1910 it was closed.[51]

To some extent, it is possible that the link with socialist idealism reduced the support which some councillors, and perhaps the Board of Education, felt that they could give to the clinic. The school clinic could be attacked in the press as a typical example of 'municipal socialism'.[52]

Clinics gained wider support through recognition of their role in the German education system. The imperial rivalry with Germany had led to increasing interest in the features of the social welfare provision believed to make a contribution to the military strength of that country. In this context, a largely medical audience was alerted to the achievements of the school clinics in Germany by the Prussophile Dr W. Leslie Mackenzie.[53] The use of the clinics became more widely known to educational audiences later, through the publication of W. H. Dawson's pamphlet on *School Doctors in Germany* in 1906, based on a study visit made in 1905.[54] In 1908 *The Times* publicized the German clinics in an extended article.[55] Both James Kerr, the head of the London County Council School Medical Service, and Newman separately visited Germany to study the clinics in action.[56]

Apart from these influences, the clinic also gained the support of the British Medical Association (BMA), which accepted the need for the treatment of schoolchildren but, for reasons already discussed, disliked the use of hospital outpatient departments. Clinics staffed by local practitioners were considered a more acceptable alternative.[57] The first clinics can be ascribed to socialist or general humanitarian impulses, both publicly funded clinics as at Bradford[58] and privately funded ventures such as the dental clinic at Cambridge.[59] They were followed by clinics founded on more pragmatic grounds. The first Welsh clinic at Abertillery was established due to the unavailability of alternative means of treatment.[60] Overall, few clinics were founded in the early years of the School Medical Service, and Newman's annual report for 1908 notes only the clinic at Bradford as being fully operational.[61]

The early clinics varied in their characteristics. Some were lavishly equipped, with full-time medical staff in attendance; others had only minimal facilities, and were dependent on the part-time, sometimes unpaid work of the local MOH or school medical officer. Most were located in school buildings or municipal offices, like the pioneer Bradford clinic, but others, especially those with some voluntary contribution involved, were housed in a variety of premises; at the dental clinic at Stanton 'a lady's drawing room is used for operations, and her garden acts as a waiting room.'[62]

By 1913 the operation of the gradually growing number of clinics had resulted in a significant output of favourable, often overtly propagandist literature supporting the concept. Typical of the literature is Lewis D. Cruickshank's work on *School Clinics at Home and Abroad*. This contains a critical appraisal of the difficulties of other means of treatment, and a series of arguments for clinics. Cruickshank saw these as having advantages in both the administration and application of treatment. Because the clinic was under the control of the education authority, problems of leakage between inspection and treatment could be minimized, delays in providing treatment reduced, attendances controlled, non-attendance monitored, and the inconvenience to parents and children alleviated.[63] Because the clinic was designed specifically to cater for the needs of schoolchildren, it could provide treatment for conditions which could not otherwise be dealt with adequately, particularly those needing frequent, continual treatment such as discharging ears. It could also offer more appropriate remedies for other conditions, including vision problems or dental defects, which went untreated or were inadequately dealt with by existing institutions. Cruickshank also argued that the clinic had social and educational advantages, helping to build up the relationship between parents, children, teachers and doctors, and connecting the local authority more closely to problems of educational hygiene.[64] Arguments for the social advantages of school meals and school clinics could be found elsewhere in the literature.

Undoubtedly the gradual but accelerating growth of school clinic provision in the years immediately preceding the First World War was aided by the advantages perceived for this type of provision. There was also the support of the BMA for a clinic system, and the refusal of some hospitals to provide treatment. Two other factors helped the spread of clinics. First, opposition to the establishment of clinics by local GPs diminished rapidly when it was seen that fears for their practices were unfounded.[65] Secondly, and more influentially, Newman gave increasing support to the concept in succeeding annual reports, leading more authorities to consider the advantages of providing clinics for both examination and treatment.[66]

Clinics were not without their disadvantages, not all of which were acknowledged by their enthusiasts. In London, some of the parents regarded the early treatment centres with distrust, and for some time public confidence in these new and unfamiliar institutions was lower than in the long-established hospital outpatient departments.[67] The scattered population in rural areas created difficulties for clinics. In Norfolk a horse-drawn caravan was used to take a mobile clinic around the schools.[68] No similar Welsh initiative is known.

Funding Treatment: Public or Private Sources?

The largely abortive provident schemes do serve to illustrate how sensitive was the question of payment for treatment provided under the School Medical Service. The 1907 Act was vague on this issue, but a subsequent Act both clarified and complicated the situation.

The Local Education Authorities (Medical Treatment) Act 1909 required education authorities to charge parents for the cost of treatment, unless the family was in necessitous circumstances.[69]

The origins of this Act lay both in an ideological desire to insist on private funding, if not private provision, and in a long-standing dispute over the division of the cost of local services between local rate and central government grant aid. The Bill originated among Moderate (Conservative) councillors on the LCC, and was introduced into Parliament by a Moderate councillor and MP, Walter Guinness. It received support from all parties, however, including among its sponsors Labour members like Ramsey MacDonald. They had been convinced by the argument that many local education authorities were diffident about using their powers under the 1907 Act because of the additional burden that would be placed on the rates.[70] As the Bill was similar in its phrasing to the Education (Provision of Meals) Act of 1906, there were also grounds for believing that the provisions for the recovery of the cost would be as ineffective as they had proved under that Act. Privately, the Board of Education was unhappy about the introduction of Guinness's Bill. Morant thought: 'the less attention we draw to the Bill so far as the public are concerned, the better.'[71] Publicly, the board felt unable to oppose its passage, accepting the arguments of its proponents in standing committee.[72] The Earl of Crewe hoped its provisions would be interpreted liberally: 'It would be very unfortunate if in any locality too hard a construction were placed upon the provision that a parent must pay if he is able to do so.'[73]

The passage of the 1909 Act created further difficulties for councils giving treatment. First, it introduced apparent anomalies and inconsistencies into the system. This was particularly the case when the voluntary hospitals were used. Parents would find on arrival at the nominated hospital that they were expected to pay for their child's treatment, even though other children under school age, and often the parents themselves, were still entitled to free treatment. In London they might already have been directed past or turned away from a hospital where the whole family had previously enjoyed free treatment. Charges increased the likelihood of parents refusing to obtain treatment, or seeking treatment from other sources.[74] Payment was often required even where parents had contributed to the Hospital Saturday Fund or similar schemes.

Some hospitals feared their subscription income would diminish as contributors felt they received poor value for their subscriptions.[75]

Second, among those councils which attempted to implement the Act fully, a cumbersome bureaucracy was required to assess cases and, where necessary, to collect charges. At a minimum, inquiries had to be made as to whether a child was necessitous, and thus eligible for free treatment, while many councils had a sliding scale of charges. This was more equitable, but also meant more comprehensive inquiries into parental circumstances. Some councils emphasized that their clinics were open only to 'children whose parents are not in a position financially (or for other reasons) to obtain treatment from other sources',[76] but this usually meant that virtually all elementary schoolchildren had access to a clinic. The LCC's scale of charges embraced all but the very highest-paid members of the working class. In this sense, the clinic was universally accessible to its elementary school clientele. Despite the apparent legal requirements imposed by the 1909 Act, there is evidence that many councils chose not to impose a charge. An LCC inquiry in 1911 found that only five out of twenty-two councils replying to a questionnaire were actually imposing charges for treatment in their clinics, and in one of these, Abertillery, no charge had in fact been levied.[77]

The failure to impose charges risked surcharge by the district auditor, but this risk was reduced by the policy of the Board of Education. As was later admitted, this was essentially to allow local authorities to make up their own minds, rather than to insist on charges being levied.[78] Correspondence with the board was actually cited as argument in favour of ignoring the requirements of the 1909 Act, and the legality of free treatment was not challenged on audit.[79] By 1918 the 1909 Act was being described as a 'dead letter' in parliamentary debate.[80] This claim was exaggerated, for in some areas considerable efforts were made to levy and collect charges for treatment. Nevertheless a survey by the board in 1921 indicates that children receiving medical treatment through the School Medical Service received such treatment free in many areas.[81] Only with the provision of spectacles, and operations for tonsils and adenoids, were more councils found to be charging than those providing treatment free. In practice, free treatment was even more widespread than these figures suggest, for seventy-one of the 210 councils claiming to charge for treatment had not received or recovered any parental contributions during the 1919–20 financial year.[82] The board therefore faced considerable opposition from the local authorities when, under pressure from the Geddes Committee to produce savings in the net cost of the School Medical Service, it attempted to force all councils to charge for treatment.[83]

Conclusions

The intervention of the School Medical Service into the lives of Welsh schoolchildren raised questions, as it did in all parts of England and Wales, about the divisions between the private world of the family and the public needs of the state. These were expressed in various arenas, not all of which are adequately documented. Families generally tolerated, indeed usually welcomed, the activity of the medical inspector, provided he did not challenge conventions too radically, and respected largely unwritten conventions about the nature of the inspection. However, in rejecting the provident model of treatment provision, they indicated that here was a role which the state was required to undertake, rather than for the family to provide for. Moreover, the inability of private medical institutions in general to deal adequately with the needs of schoolchildren – and the needs of the parents who accompanied them – was one of the factors encouraging the growth of a publicly provided school clinic system.

Notes

[1] Education (Provision of Meals) Act 1906 (6 Edw. VII, c. 57); Education (Administrative Provisions) Act 1907 (7 Edw. VII, c. 43); Children Act 1908 (8 Edw. VII, c. 67).

[2] The titles of many of the earlier histories of welfare reflect this emphasis; for example Fraser, D. (1973), *The Evolution of the British Welfare State* (London, Macmillan).

[3] See Finlayson, G. (1990), 'A moving frontier: voluntarism and the state in British social welfare 1941–49', *Twentieth Century British History*, 1, 2, 183–206; Whiteside, N. (1983), 'Private agencies for public purposes: some new perspectives on policy making in health insurance between the wars', *Journal of Social Policy*, 12, 165–93; Kidd, A. (1999), *State, Society and the Poor in Nineteenth Century England* (Basingstoke, Macmillan).

[4] Klein, R. and O'Higgins, M. (eds) (1985), *The Future of Welfare* (Oxford, Blackwell), p. 133.

[5] See BPP 1904/XXXII:1, *Report of the Inter-Departmental Committee on Physical Deterioration*, Cd. 2175, 1904.

[6] Mackenzie, W. L. (1904), *The Medical Inspection of School Children* (Edinburgh and Glasgow, Wm. Hodge & Co.), p. 76.

[7] See e.g. BPP 1895/XLVII:1, *Royal Commission on Secondary Education*, vol. 5: *Memoranda and Answers to Questions*, C. 7862-iv, pp. 352–5, and Hendrick, H., 'Child labour, medical capital and the school medical service c.1890–1918', in Cooter, R. (ed.) (1992), *In the Name of the Child: Health and Welfare 1880–1940* (London, Routledge), pp. 45–71

[8] Hirst, J. D. (1991), 'Public health and the public elementary schools, 1870–1907', *History of Education*, 20, 107–18.

[9] Harris, B. (1995), *The Health of the Schoolchild* (Buckingham, Open University Press).

[10] See Markham, V. (1956), *Friendship's Harvest* (London, Reinhardt) and Webster, C. (1982), 'Healthy or hungry thirties', *History Workshop*, 13, 100–29.

[11] *Lancet*, ii (1908), 208.

[12] *School Hygiene*, 1 (1910), 667.

[13] PRO Ed 23/201, memorandum, Selby-Bigge to Morant, 22 December 1908; *Lancet*, i (1909), 914; *Medical Officer*, 1 (1909), 851–6.

[14] West Ham CBC, *Annual Report of the School Medical Officer for 1908*, p. 14.

[15] *Lancet*, i (1912), 59.

[16] Carmarthenshire CC, *Annual Report of the School Medical Officer for 1911*, p. 11.

[17] Carmarthenshire CC, *Annual Report of the School Medical Officer for 1908*, p. 4. For a general discussion on the difficulties of early statistical returns, see Hirst, D., 'A note on early school medical service statistics', *Local Population Studies*, 44 (1990), 60–2.

[18] Carmarthenshire CC, *Annual Report of the School Medical Officer for 1913*, pp. 5–6; PRO, Ed 50/35, memorandum on areas where the MOH is not SMO, dated 1922.

[19] Gilbert, B. B. (1966), *The Evolution of National Insurance in Great Britain: The Origins of the Welfare State* (London, Michael Joseph), pp. 129–30; Hirst, J. D. (1989), 'The growth of treatment through the School Medical Service, 1908–18', *Medical History*, 33, 318–42; Daglish, N. D. (1990), 'Robert Morant's hidden agenda? The origins of the medical treatment of children', *History of Education*, 19, 139–48.

[20] PRO Ed 50/5, Circular 576, full preliminary draft.

[21] Ibid.

[22] PRO Ed 24/280, Morant to Newman, 15 November 1907.

[23] Board of Education, *Memorandum on Medical Inspection of Children in Public Elementary Schools*, Circular 576/1907, paras 14 and 15.

[24] Board of Education, *Circular to Local Authorities under Part III of the Education Act, 1902, on Certain Questions arising under Section Thirteen of the Education (Administrative Provisions) Act 1907*, Circular 596/1908, 17 August 1908.

[25] PRO Ed 50/7, memorandum by Newman, 29 June 1908.

[26] Ibid.

[27] *Lancet*, i (1910), 1294.

[28] Cruickshank, L. D. (1913), *School Clinics: At Home and Abroad* (London, National League for Physical Education and Improvement), pp. 38–9.

[29] Denbighshire CC School Children Sub-Committee minutes, 6 October 1909.

[30] BPP 1910/XXIII:1, Board of Education, *Annual Report of the Chief Medical Officer for 1908*, Cd. 4986, p. 34.

[31] See Davey, I. (1913), *School Clinics as a Means of Providing Medical Aid to School Children* (Guildford, n.p.); Newsholme, A. (1931), *International Studies on the Relation between the Private and the Official Practice of Medicine*, vol. 3 (London, George Allen & Unwin), pp. 367–76.

[32] *Lancet*, ii (1911), 347–9.

[33] LCC, Education Committee, minutes, 26 June 1907.

[34] Remmett Weaver, A. E. (1911), 'The Abertillery school clinic', *School Hygiene*, 2, 522.

[35] For a discussion on deterrence and other forms of rationing in social policy, see Parker, R. A., 'Social administration and scarcity', in Butterworth, E. and Holmans, R. (eds) (1975), *Social Welfare in Modern Britain* (London, Fontana).

[36] Shropshire CC, *Annual Report of the School Medical Officer for 1915*, p. 11.

[37] See BPP 1910/XXIII:175, Board of Education, *Annual Report of the Chief Medical Officer for 1909*, Cd. 5426, pp. 198–202; BPP 1911/XVII:449, Board of Education, *Annual Report of the Chief Medical Officer for 1910*, Cd. 5925, pp. 270–6; BPP 1912–13/XXI:439, Board of Education, *Annual Report of the Chief Medical Officer for 1911*, Cd. 6530, pp. 290–301.

[38] West Bromwich CBC, *Annual Report of the School Medical Officer for 1912*, p. 8.

[39] See e.g. *The Times*, 1 September 1908, p. 8.

[40] See Hirst, J. D. (1981), 'A failure without parallel: the School Medical Service and the London County Council, 1907–1912', *Medical History*, 25, 281–300. For Margaret McMillan see Lowndes, G. A. N. (1960), *Margaret McMillan: The Children's Champion* (London, Museum Press); Bradburn, E. (1989), *Margaret McMillan: Portrait of a Pioneer* (London, Routledge); Steedman, C. (1990) *Childhood, Culture and Class in Britain: Margaret McMillan, 1860–1931* (New Brunswick, Rutgers University Press).

[41] LCC Education Committee, agenda, 9 December 1908, p. 114.

[42] Derbyshire CC, *Annual Report of the School Medical Officer for 1909*, p. 45.

[43] Gwynedd RO, Caernarfon, Carnarvon CC, School Attendance and Medical Inspection Sub-Committee, minutes, 28 September 1911.

[44] PRO Ed 125/8, Precedent Cover: Carnarvon.

[45] Gwynedd RO, Caernarfon, Bontnewydd school medical relief fund account book, 1911–14.

[46] Gwynedd RO, Caernarfon, School Attendance and Medical Inspection Sub-Committee, minutes, 21 November 1911.

[47] Ibid., 25 January 1912.

[48] Carnarvonshire County Council, *Annual Report of the School Medical Officer for 1912*, p. 11.

[49] For details of the grant system and calculations, see PRO Ed 50/63, Medical Department procedure minute M27.

[50] *Justice*, 10 March 1906.

[51] See McMillan, M. (1927), *The Life of Rachel McMillan* (London, J. M. Dent & Sons), p. 118.

[52] *The Times*, 1 September 1908, 8.

[53] Mackenzie, W. L. (1906), *The Health of the School Child* (London, Methuen & Co.).

[54] Dawson, W. H. (1906), *School Doctors in Germany*, Board of Education, Educational Pamphlets, 4 (London, Wyman & Sons for HMSO).

[55] *The Times*, 23 August 1908, p. 11.

[56] PRO MH 139/1, Newman diaries, vol. 1, 10–25 March 1909.

[57] *British Medical Journal*, ii (1908), supplement, 42.

[58] McMillan, M. (1909), *New Life in Our Schools* (Manchester, Women's Co-operative Guild), p. 5.

[59] *School Hygiene*, 1 (1910), p. 247.

[60] Remmett Weaver, 'The Abertillery school clinic', 514–22.

[61] BPP 1910/XXIII:1, p. 97.

[62] Cruickshank, *School Clinics*, pp. 130–1.

[63] Ibid., p. 60.

[64] Ibid., pp. 58–9.

[65] *School Hygiene*, 1 (1910), 522.

[66] See BPP 1911/XVII:449, pp. 139, 146–65; BPP 1912–13/XXI:439, pp. 132–47; BPP 1914/XXV:401, Board of Education, *Annual Report of the Chief Medical Officer for 1912*, Cd. 7184, pp. 166–85.

[67] LCC, Children's Care (Central) Sub-Committee, agenda, 30 May 1913.

[68] BPP 1914–16/XVIII:665, Board of Education, *Annual Report of the Chief Medical Officer for 1914*, Cd. 8055, p. 123.

[69] Local Education Authorities (Medical Treatment) Act 1909 (9 Edw. VII, c. 13).

[70] *Parl. Deb.* (Lords), 5th series, 2 (29 July 1909), col. 842.

[71] PRO Ed 50/3, written footnote to memorandum on the 1909 Act.

[72] *The Times*, 19 May 1909, 4.

[73] *Parl. Deb.* (Lords), 5th series, 2 (29 July 1909), col. 843.

[74] *Lancet*, ii (1910), 1437.

[75] LCC, Children's Care (Central) Sub-Committee, agenda, 27 January 1911.

[76] Wigan CBC, *Annual Report of the School Medical Officer for 1909*, p. 19.

[77] LCC, Children's Care (Central) Sub-Committee, agenda, 27 January 1911.

[78] PRO Ed 50/66, minute on 'charges for treatment', 15 March 1923.

[79] *Medical Officer*, 11 (1914), 74.

[80] *Parl. Deb.* (Commons), 5th series, 104 (18 March 1918), col. 703.

[81] PRO Ed 50/60, charges for treatment, 1919–20.

[82] Ibid. In some cases, as with the prescription of glasses, the charge could be a direct transaction between parents and optician, which would not be shown in the accounts.

[83] PRO Ed 50/66, minute on 'charges for treatment', 15 March 1923.

5

A Proletarian Public Sphere: Working-Class Provision of Medical Services and Care in South Wales, c.1900–1948[1]

STEVEN THOMPSON

Introduction

This chapter considers the existence of a proletarian public sphere in the first half of the twentieth century in south Wales, through an examination of working-class provision of medical attendance. Two concepts were central to Habermas's formulation of the bourgeois public sphere. Firstly, he stressed the importance of 'rational, critical debate' as a constitutive feature of the public sphere.[2] Participation in debate in matters of concern was not determined by the status or identity of the proponent of an argument but was predicated on the 'force of the better argument'. Rational discourse embodying universal truths and reason gave the public sphere its essential shape and negated biases of time, culture or power.[3] The second fundamental feature of the public sphere, deriving from the first, was its openness to popular participation. The institutions of the public sphere formed a 'forum of discursive interaction that was ostensibly open and accessible to all, where private citizens could discuss matters of public interest freely, rationally and as equals'.[4] Every individual was able to engage in debate in the public sphere.

Habermas's conception of the public sphere has proven very controversial. Most critics have attacked Habermas's rather idealized conception of the inclusiveness of the bourgeois public sphere.[5] Marxists have stressed his neglect of working-class

movements, feminist critiques object to his lack of any consideration of gender and others have criticized his idea of 'rational'
debate.[6] Most relevant to this chapter are those studies that have
posited an alternative or counter-public, situated in the associ-
ational worlds of working-class people. This chapter discusses the
provision of medical attendance in south Wales in light of these
studies of proletarian public spheres.[7]

Club Practice in South Wales

Before the creation of the National Health Service (NHS) in 1948,
working-class people obtained medical attendance and care by a
variety of means. They utilized philanthropic institutions and a
variety of insurance systems to gain access to medical treatment
during times of illness.[8] Notable among working-class efforts were
the works clubs whereby workers arranged with their employer for
an agreed sum to be deducted from their pay and for a doctor to be
appointed from the accumulated total.[9] Known more commonly in
south Wales as medical aid societies, they provided medical attendance and drugs for the workmen and their dependants in return for
a payment of about 2d or 3d in each pound of the workers' wages.
Workers contributed when they were healthy and employed, and
received sick benefits and medical attendance when they were ill. In
a similar fashion, many groups of workers organized for a deduc-
tion to be made from their wages for cottage hospitals to be built
and maintained, or else arranged for this through their medical aid
societies.

The services provided by these societies were intended as
comprehensive public services – public in the sense that they were
accessible to as large a number of people as possible. Initially begun
as works clubs in the late nineteenth and early twentieth centuries,
many of the more active societies had by the inter-war period evolved
to become sophisticated organizations providing medical attendance
and a host of other services to the whole community in which they
were situated. While many schemes were connected to a certain
place of work, and limited to the workers employed there, others
attempted to increase the number of members they possessed.
Higher revenues meant a better-developed and more comprehensive
service, and so it was common for committees to approach and

welcome additional groups of workers to their schemes and make
the schemes as universal as possible. In addition, many schemes
allowed workers to provide medical attendance for their families. A
typical example of these larger, more inclusive societies was the
Tredegar Medical Aid Society.[10] Begun in 1874 by a section of the
miners and steelworkers of the town, the society gradually developed
into a much more ambitious and comprehensive scheme, so that by
the 1920s about 95 per cent of the population of the town were
eligible for medical treatment from the society.[11] The miners and
steelworkers paid according to a poundage system of deductions of
2d in each pound of their weekly wages, while so-called 'town
subscribers' paid 18s per year directly to the society. Similarly, the
Ebbw Vale Workmen's Medical Society provided medical attendance
and benefit for 24,000 people by 1920, while the Llanelli and District
Medical Service had about 18,100 subscribers in August 1937, which,
if dependants were taken into account, meant that about 54,000
were covered for medical services by this society.[12]

Therefore, although eligibility was based upon the payment of a
subscription, these schemes established by a section of the workforce became, in many cases, a public service as efforts were made
to make them accessible to large proportions of the population.
The workmen who dominated the management of these societies
made repeated efforts to make them as inclusive as possible. Aged
workmen and widows were able to call on the Tredegar society's
services at no charge, while other societies successfully made
provision for the unemployed during the Depression of the inter-
war years.[13] In these ways, the medical aid societies of south Wales
were an articulation not only of an individualized notion of self-
help, but also of a collectivized mutuality that made the sick and
the ill a charge on the whole community. As one subscriber commented, 'Now we one help the other, and hundreds and hundreds
there are who, if they did not club together in this kind of way,
would never be able to get any doctor at all.'[14]

'Those who Pay the Piper should Call the Tune':[15] Control of Club Practices

A crucial aspect of the medical aid societies was the struggle for
financial control waged between the workmen and their represent-

atives on the one hand, and the medical establishment and employers on the other. During the nineteenth century, the tendency was for employers to collect deductions from their employees' wages and pay a doctor or surgeon from the accumulated total. Employers often had the power to appoint and dismiss doctors and had a close relationship with the doctors as a result.[16] This became increasingly unpopular with the workmen, especially after the passing of the Workmen's Compensation Act of 1897. It seemed to the workmen that the doctors obeyed the instructions of employers and were inclined to give testimony favourable to the employers in compensation cases that came before the local courts.[17]

Rather than have the colliery companies collect the dues from the men and hand them over to the doctors, financial control was acquired by workmen's funds in many cases and doctors were paid set salaries.[18] The last few years of the nineteenth century and the first decade of the twentieth were characterized by a significant level of agitation and controversy as workmen's committees attempted to wrest control of the schemes from the employers. Workmen in many places successfully gained control, and it was this lay control that most provoked the anger of the British Medical Association (BMA) and the medical establishment.[19] But it is clear that, for their part, workmen and their committees considered lay control to be an integral part of their efforts to provide a comprehensive public service for their communities. Workmen's committees considered themselves the disinterested protectors of the 'public good' against the selfish, egotistical interests of the medical profession and acquired control so as to put funds to the best public use.[20] The profit motive was supplanted and excess funds used further to develop services.

Reformers argued that if doctors were appointed on set salaries the money that remained from the weekly deductions could be used to build libraries or workmen's institutes, or even clear the debts of the Miners' Federation.[21] Others focused on the development of medical services and argued that the money could be used to provide nurses, more assistants, bone-setters, better-qualified doctors, medical appliances such as artificial limbs, and more comfortable surgeries. One such reformer even argued that doctors 'would have more time to devote to their cases, will take keener interest in their noble mission, keep in closer touch with results of modern research' and would be motivated not by 'the pecuniary advantages which the farming of colliery paradises afford' but by more genuine aspirations.[22] In September 1904, representatives of the Aberaman and District Workmen's Doctors Fund set out their reasons for trying to wrest control from their employers and in doing so invoked the notion of action for the 'public good'. They stated:

> we are confident that with the enormous sums of money contributed by us annually, we can secure a better system of medical aid . . . We can also maintain a Cottage Hospital in our district, with all its benefits, and we ask why should selfish and personal 'greed for gold' endeavour to prevent the great principle of the 'greatest good for the greatest number'.[23]

The workers of other districts similarly hoped to establish cottage hospitals and many were successful in achieving this aim. A short period after gaining financial control of their club practice, the workers of Rhymney opened a cottage hospital equipped with twelve beds. 'A more honourable testimony to the forethought and prudence of our colliery workmen it would be difficult to adduce,' opined Polonius, the editorialist of the *Merthyr Express*. 'All honour to the Rhymney workmen,' he added.[24] The cottage hospitals at Ebbw Vale, Tredegar, Abertysswg and Blaina were similarly established through the efforts of the medical aid societies situated in those places.

Therefore, workers in south Wales held definite ideas as to what they thought their medical services should be and took measures to implement these ideas. They envisaged a public service organized upon the principle of the 'greatest good for the greatest number' and fought the medical establishment to establish these services. Although the 1911 National Health Insurance Act curtailed the expansion of these medical aid societies it did not completely emasculate them. Small improvements continued to be made so that by the inter-war period the schemes of south Wales were among the most sophisticated and highly developed club practices in the whole of Britain. To take Tredegar as an example once more, by the 1920s the society offered its members the services of five doctors, one surgeon, two pharmacists, a physiotherapist, a dentist and a district nurse. For an additional 4d a week, members were covered for hospital treatment, and a car was provided to the railway station where a first-class ticket was made available to reach the hospital. Glasses could be obtained for 2s 6d, while false teeth were sold at less than cost price. Artificial limbs, injections, patent foods, drugs, X-rays and even wigs were all free to members.[25] Similarly, the Llanelli and District Medical Service offered its members a general practitioner service, ophthalmic, ear, nose, throat and general surgery services, and defrayed the cost of special drugs.[26]

A Proletarian Public Sphere

The creation and administration of these medical services was carried out within a proletarian public sphere.[27] Firstly, the committees that administered them were run on democratic principles. While initially administered by industrialists or managers of the local collieries, the societies came increasingly to be controlled by workmen's committees.[28] The powers of these committees varied from one scheme to the next – some only had the power to appoint or dismiss a doctor while others were able to discipline a doctor's conduct and regulate his working arrangements. The tendency, however, was for these committees to assume more extensive responsibilities in the late nineteenth and early twentieth centuries. Appointment to these committees was by ballot of the members but it would be wrong to assume that this was merely representative democracy in action, for it was very much participatory in nature. In many cases, important decisions facing a committee were put to a ballot of the members.[29] Thus a ballot of the workmen was taken to appoint a chief doctor for the Tredegar society in March 1911,[30] while a public meeting was similarly held by the Bedlinog Medical Committee in June 1922 to vote on the appointment of another doctor. In this latter case the applications and testimonials of each applicant were read out and 1,000 voting papers distributed to subscribers (Figure 5.1).[31]

An applicant for a position with the Dowlais Workers' Medical Fund in 1913 was obliged to appear before a packed public meeting of over 400 people and speak at length about his career, including his experiences during the Boer War, his good relationship with his current patients in Pontyberem, and his almost total abstinence from alcohol.[32] Similarly, public meetings were held during the

inter-war years to ask certain workmen to increase their contributions to aid societies in that difficult period,[33] and meetings of the
unemployed were also held to discuss their relationship with the
societies.[34]

In any mass meeting of colliers or other workmen in south
Wales, the usual practice was for anybody who had something to
say to stand up and make their comment. Debate was open to
anyone with anything to express on a particular matter regardless
of position or status.[35] Furthermore, oratory at these public
meetings involved an interactive relationship between speaker and
audience that ensured that the opinions and feelings of society
members were clearly expressed. Newspaper reports of meetings
show that speakers were constantly being interrupted with cries of
approval or objection from those present, so that even usually
inarticulate groups and individuals could make their feelings felt in
a very direct way and play some part in determining actions and
policies.[36] Nor was this the only way in which ordinary people
could enter the realm of public debate. In a dispute between the
committee of the Llanelli and District Medical Service and their
doctors lasting almost two years, numerous letters were regularly
published in the local newspapers representing all shades of
opinion, including the doctors, the workmen's committee, the
BMA, the Socialist Medical Association and, most importantly,
members of the scheme.[37]

The debate that resulted was informed and knowledgeable in the
sense that it emanated directly from the everyday experiences of
working-class people. This was demonstrated by a reorganization
of the fund of the Nixon's collieries' workmen in Mountain Ash in
June 1904. The committee wanted to reorganize the scheme so as
to engage doctors directly and place them under their control. A
detailed plan was drawn up and presented to a meeting of the
workmen for consideration but, after full discussion and a ballot,
the workmen rejected the scheme. Instead, amendments and
additions to the old medical fund rules were passed which
included: provision that doctors ensure that another doctor be
on call if a patient's particular doctor was unavailable; that
doctors provide and pay for all specialists when required; that
dispensers be kept in all dispensaries, four hours in the morning and four hours in the evening; and that doctors be required
to provide rooms for the assistants to sleep in the surgeries at

Tredegar Workmen's Medical Aid and Sick Relief Fund.

APPOINTMENT OF CHIEF MEDICAL OFFICER.

To the Members,

In accordance with the Resolution passed at a Public Meeting, held at the Town Hall, Tredegar, on Saturday, February 4th, 1911,

A BALLOT

to select a Chief Medical Officer will take place on Friday next, February 10th, 1911; to be conducted at the Works and Colliery.

At the request of the above Meeting Councillor A. Onions, J.P., Miners' Agent, gave particulars of each Candidate interviewed, and briefly stated the opinion of the Committee on each, who placed them in order of Merit as follows :—

1. DR. E. T. H. DAVIES, M.D., Lond.; M.S., Lond.; F.R.C.S., Eng.;

2. DR. J. W. GLENTON-MYLER, F.R.C.S., Eng.; L.R.C.P., Lond.; D.P.H.; M.D., Brussels;

3. DR. T. E. FRANCIS, M.D.; B.S.; D.P.H.; all Lond.

In reference to each of above Candidates Mr. Onions stated that Dr. Davies held the highest Degrees obtainable in England, and gave it as his opinion that he was a man of high business abilities and well fitted for the post.

Dr. Glenton-Myler was also an excellent Candidate who had high Qualifications and has had much experience—especially in India.

Dr. Francis also has excellent Qualifications and is a young man of promising ability.

The above remarks do not apply to the present Staff, or to Dr. H. G. Brown, or Dr. J. O. D. Wade, Cardiff; as the Committee are of opinion that they are all well-known to the Members who will therefore be able to judge for themselves.

The Ballot Paper will be in the following form and each Member is requested to

VOTE FOR ONE CANDIDATE ONLY.

Please place your X opposite the Candidate you desire to vote for.

No Person under 16 years of age will be allowed to vote.

BALLOT PAPER.

No.	NAME.	QALIFICATIONS.
1	BARBER, A.	M.B., B.S., M.R.C.S., L.R.C.P., D.P.H., Lond
2	BROWN, HORACE G.	M.R.C.S., Eng., L.R.C.P., Lond., B.A., Camb.
3	CCLYER, S.	M.D., B.S., Lond., M.R.C.P., Lond., D.P.H., Camb.
4	COUMBE, J. BATTEN	M.D., F.R.C.S., Eng., L.S.A., Lond., D.P.H., Oxon.
5	CRAWFORD, I.	L.R.C.P., M.R.C.S., L.F.P.S.
6	DAVIES, E. T. H.	M.D., Lond., M.S., Lond., F.R.C.S., Eng.
7	FRANCIS, T. E.	M.D., B.S., D.P.H., all Lond.
8	GLENTON-MYLER, J. W.	F.R.C.S. Eng., L.R.C.P., Lond., D.P.H.,M.D., Brussels.
9	ROBERTSON, ALEX.	M.B., M.S., Edinburgh
10	STONEY, G. F.	L.R.C.P., L.F.P.S., all Edinburgh and Glasgow
11	WADE, J. O. D.	M.B., Lond., B.S. Lond., M.R.C.S., Eng., L.R.C.P., Lond.
12	WISE, ROBERT	M.D., M.B., C.M.

Please place a **X** opposite the name of the person you intend to vote for.

Definitions of Qualifcations.

M.D.	Doctor of Medicine (Highest Degree possible in Medicine)	M.S.	Master of Surgery
M.B.	Bachelor of Medicine	B.S.	Bachelor of Surgery
L.R.C.P.	Licentiate Royal College Physicians	M.R.C.S.	Member Royal College of Surgeons
M.R.C.P.	Member Royal College Physicians	L.F.P.S.	Licentiate Royal Faculty of Physicians and Surgeons
D.P.H.	Diploma Public Health	L.S.A.	Licentiate of Associated Surgeons
F.R.C.S.	Fellow Royal College of Surgeons (Highest Degree possible in Surgery)		

Signed on behalf of the General Committee.

WALTER ONIONS, Chairman
A. S. TALLIS, Trustee
S. FILER, Trustee
T. P. BAINES, Trustee
ALFRED ONIONS, Miners' Agent
JNO. LLOYD

W. CONWAY
THOS. PEARCE
RICHARD M. CHILDS
ELLIS LEWIS
THOS. DAVIES
JAS. STRADLING

JOHN PRICE
SAMUEL PHILLIPS
JAS. WILLIAMS
DAN ROBERTS
WM. MORGAN
ALFRED DAVIES

J. L. HERBERT, Gen. Sec.

Swarbrick, Printer, Tredegar.

Figure 5.1 Poster advertising a meeting to elect the chief medical officer of the Tredegar Medical Aid Society (Gwent Record Office)[38]

night.[39] But debate was not only experientially informed, for the members of the various schemes were kept briefed by the officials and doctors, especially when disputes between them broke out. In one such dispute in Mountain Ash in 1913 a 'kind of duel with handbills' took place as each side put its case,[40] while in a similar dispute in Llanelli in 1934 the air was said to be thick with manifestos and counter-manifestos.[41]

Therefore, the medical aid societies of south Wales constituted a service in which a democratic polity exercised power. A 'public' was able to express itself through its arrangements for medical treatment and a space was created characterized by those vital aspects of Habermas's bourgeois public sphere – popular participation and informed debate. The internal world of organized labour constituted a participatory proletarian public sphere within which discourse was tempered by experience of everyday reality and from which an emancipatory language was projected as a challenge to the medical establishment and the bourgeois hegemony.

However, the democratic nature of these 'subscriber democracies' should not be idealized and there were a number of factors that served to impair the essential form of the public sphere. Firstly, complaints were occasionally voiced that the committees that administered the club practices were undemocratic. Alfred Cox of the BMA, in an address to the Monmouthshire Division in July 1920, attacked the committees that were making 'wage slaves' of the doctors of that part of south Wales. He maintained:

> nobody can pretend that workmen's committees as you know them in this part of the country are comparable as responsible bodies to publicly elected authorities subject to central government, audit, and supervision, and open to the criticism, of public opinion. You know too much of the way in which such committees are formed; the artificial and artful way in which the supposed demand is worked up; the 'mass meetings,' often consisting of 2 or 3 per cent. of the workmen concerned, which are announced as having agreed to a 'medical scheme'; the farcical 'ballots'; the combination of apathy on the one hand and trade union pressure on the other which together lead many who would willingly have stayed with their old doctor to fall in with the agitators and pay to the new doctor rather than seem 'disloyal to the union'. These things are commonplace to you, but they are happily almost unknown to your colleagues in industrial and colliery practice outside Wales.[42]

Cox stated that doctors did not mind taking service under town councils, insurance committees or Poor Law guardians because these were '*publicly* elected bodies with a sense of *public* responsibility, kept in check by *public* criticism' (my emphasis). Committees of workmen, he asserted, met none of these criteria.[43]

Cox was clearly and predictably antipathetic to the lay control of medical services, but at times other individuals were similarly dissatisfied with the administration of these services. A subscriber to the Abertysswg and Rhymney McLaren Collieries Doctors' Fund complained in 1903, for example, that meetings of the committee established to administer the fund were rarely held, that the few meetings that were held were purposely held at inconvenient times so as to prevent debate and that meetings were 'rushed' by certain members or groups on the committee to ensure their interests were served. The committee, he claimed, was not democratic but more akin to a 'Mutual Admiration Society' as members ensured that only friends were elected. He further alleged that balance sheets were not produced, the rule that sitting committee members should retire after certain periods of time was ignored, committee members were paid large amounts of money in expenses, and rules were drawn up or struck out without consultation with the workmen.[44]

However, criticisms of the democratic nature of club practices by their members were rare. More significantly, the decisions taken by the committees administering such schemes were not always as consensual as they might have been and seem to have derived from the determination of more ideologically committed members of the labour movement to advance their cause. Class-conscious members of the labour movement attempted to assert working-class aims over the aims of other groups in their communities but often came up against the apathy of their fellow workers or the enduring appeal of 'community' as opposed to 'class' in the political consciousness of their fellow workers.[45] For example, when the committee of the Abertridwr workmen attempted to set up a rival medical aid society to challenge the old system in 1920, they provoked a split in the ranks of the workmen and were only able to entice less than half the men to their new scheme.[46] More significantly, the dispute in Llanelli also caused a split in the workmen with more than half staying loyal to the old doctors and only a minority enlisting with the Llanelli Workmen's Committee's new scheme. In this latter case, a large group of workmen remained on the lists of the old doctors and accused the official Workmen's Medical Committee of being unrepresentative and of acting unconstitutionally.[47]

There were also instances, especially during the Edwardian period, when debate and discussion in the proletarian sphere, far from being rational, was highly partisan in character. A class-conscious and oppositional language was used in the struggles over control of the club practices as the more ideologically 'advanced' members of the labour movement fought for greater working-class control. The older works clubs, where doctors received the total sum from the weekly deductions of the workers and were appointed by the employers, were described as 'exploitative', 'tyrannical', 'extortionate' and 'oppressive', and the workers were said to exist in 'bondage' and 'slavery'.[48] Those who opposed these arrangements and advocated a reform of the system argued that they sought 'justice', 'liberty', 'freedom', 'emancipation', 'salvation', 'respect' and 'equality'.[49] One letter advocating workers' control of medical attendance at Merthyr, signed 'Llef Cyfiawnder' ('Cry for justice'), ended with the exhortation 'Weithwyr Dowlais, byddwch yn ddynion rhydd' ('Workers of Dowlais, be free men').[50]

Therefore, notions of 'justice', 'liberty', 'freedom' and 'equality' were invoked in order to assert working-class rights over the rights of other classes. Furthermore, proletarian discourse was not 'rational' in the sense that it was occasionally coercive and combative. In the Nixon's Collieries dispute of 1913, a workers' representative advised the men to 'fight hard' against the doctors who had treated them without respect and who were thus undeserving of any respect themselves.[51] Similarly the Aberaman and District Workmen's Doctors Fund issued a statement in 1904 advising the doctors in their area that if they wanted 'peace' then all would be well, 'But should they court war, well then, the Welsh workman knows how to fight.'[52]

The best example of this coercive language was in the conflict between the Llanelli and District Workmen's Committee and its doctors in 1934–5. Accusations and recriminations were traded by the workmen's committee and the doctors in an atmosphere that the *Llanelly Mercury* described as 'sordid'.[53] 'Principles have been ousted by personalities', it declared, and maintained that the dispute was 'an insult to the high standards of the medical profession, the soundest principles of trade unionism and collective bargaining, and high ideals which we all have been taught to cherish'.[54] Rather than 'rational, critical debate', the exchange between the two sides consisted of attacks on each other's position and statements. As the *Llanelly Mercury* asserted: 'So confusing have been the "bulletins", that many people have been at a loss where to bestow their allegiance. Apparently authoritative statements appear to clash in their definition of fact, leaving the reader in a state of bewilderment.'[55] The statements made by each side in the newspapers seem to be attempts to gain acclamation for stances adopted and actions already taken.

Therefore, discussion in the proletarian public sphere, rather than being 'rational', was often a dramatic and exhortative battle-cry couched in a bloody-minded and violent language. Appeals to a

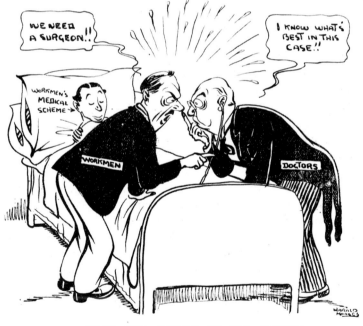

WHAT WILL HAPPEN TO THE PATIENT?

Figure 5.2 'What will happen to the patient?' This cartoon, published in March 1934, characterizes the dispute in Llanelli as a disagreement over the scheme between the workmen and the doctors. (*Llanelly Star*)[56]

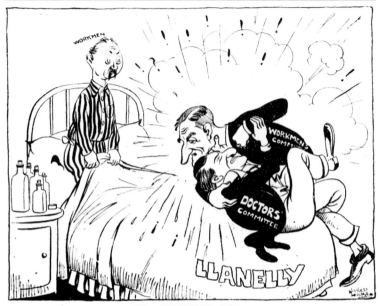

NO ARMISTICE YET.

Figure 5.3 'No Armistice yet.' This second cartoon, published in October 1934, provides an interesting insight into the nature of the dispute in Llanelli. The dispute had deteriorated into a fractious disagreement between committees as the workmen were left as bystanders. (*Llanelly Star*)[57]

universal, rational 'truth' were made, but, when necessary, a more oppositional language was used. The language used by these 'reformers' demonstrates that these attempts to gain control of the systems of medical attendance must be understood as part of a wider, emancipatory struggle on the part of the more ideologically informed sections of the labour movement in south Wales.[58] They can be seen as an attempt to provoke the working class in the Valley communities into action and an effort to arouse greater class-consciousness.[59] Workmen were encouraged to think of their own interests as being opposed to the interests of employers and the medical establishment.

Finally, and perhaps most importantly, the proletarian public sphere was, like other 'publics', a public that in defining itself excluded certain sections of the community. The proletarian public sphere of south Wales was very much gendered in nature. Certainly women had a part to play in supporting the hospitals set up by the men of their communities. Some acted as collectors or helped in fund-raising during the Hospital weeks and carnivals, while other groups of women formed themselves into 'linen leagues' to cut bandages.[60] Crucially, however, the only women involved in the public sphere, where matters of concern were discussed and decisions taken, were the 'women worthies' of a locality who obtained representation on the management committees by virtue of their husbands' contributions.[61]

In contrast, no women sat on the committees administering the medical aid societies. Obtaining the vast bulk of their finances from workmen at their place of employment, the medical aid societies were consequently controlled by these same workmen. Representatives of collieries or metalworks were elected by the workmen from amongst their ranks[62] or by the directors of the companies. Furthermore, many of the mass public meetings held to discuss the business of the societies were held either at the place of employment or else as part of trade union meetings, and women were thus unlikely to attend. Most women and children were covered for medical attendance under these schemes by virtue of the deductions made from their husbands' and fathers' pay packets, and this payment allowed the men participation in the administration of the schemes. At a meeting of the Neath and District Medical Aid Society at the end of 1938, the chairman informed those present that the matter to be discussed was for members only, and not dependants, and asked all non-members to leave the meeting. This was met with immediate uproar and the meeting degenerated into a noisy and unproductive affair.[63]

This exclusion of women in south Wales from the management and control of medical aid societies provoked a letter to the *Caerphilly Journal* in 1920 at the time of a dispute between the workmen and doctors of Abertridwr over financial control.[64] Signed 'Mothers of Abertridwr', the letter urged the men to stay faithful to the 'skilful, manly and sober' doctors who had served them so selflessly over the years, as opposed to the 'stiff, curt' men that the unfamiliar newcomers would undoubtedly be. This remarkable letter is rather sycophantic in tone and would have served the doctors' case very well, leading to doubts about its authenticity, but what is most interesting about it is the recognition that it gives to women's lack of involvement in the committee and the assertion that women were central to the processes of caring and treating illness and sickness in the family:

What a cry there has been for votes for women. Where are our votes today in regard to the present question? We mothers want to know why we have not a vote, or voice, in this, of such great importance to us? All mothers want to speak on the subject, but their cry is, Where shall we? Every advantage is given us on other elections, Council, etc., and we are urged there by any means, why not on this occasion? It is the mothers know whom they want to attend to themselves and children. Husbands, brothers and sons, consider, we want a good word in this matter. You consult us on all other subjects, why not this? Whichever way it goes, we will be women and have our own doctors after all. It is we that know the worth of the right man in the right place. It is mothers that see the smiles of their delicate suffering darlings when they see the family doctor come in that has attended to them ever since life was given.[65]

When participation in the public sphere was predicated on paid employment, the women of south Wales were inevitably to be excluded from participation in debate and discussion.

An Alternative Culture?

The nature of the proletarian public sphere in south Wales ties in with the distinctive historiographical debate, initiated by Dai Smith and Hywel Francis and taken up more recently by Chris Williams, concerning the emergence of an 'alternative culture' in south Wales that rejected the social, political and cultural norms of the bourgeois, Liberal hegemony.[66] Smith and Francis locate the emergence of this 'alternative culture' in the years 1925 and 1926. But in regard to the, albeit more narrowly defined, area of medical services, a case can perhaps be made for an earlier emergence of a rejectionist discourse. The medical aid societies of south Wales involved the rejection of professional control of medical services (and indeed over specialized knowledge), the profit motive that characterized professional control and the very idea of individualism.

Raymond Williams has written about hegemony and alternative cultures, and has distinguished between *incorporated* and *oppositional* alternative cultures.[67] The extent to which this alternative culture was also oppositional varied in time and extent and from one place to another, but clearly the conflicts between men and doctors over control of the societies involved diametrically opposed beliefs as to how the services should be organized. However, care must be taken not to exaggerate the alternative and oppositional nature of this culture and it is important to recognize that in many instancēs when 'alternative' strategies were advocated, there were individuals and groups within the proletarian sphere willing to defend the bourgeois, Liberal status quo, leading to divisions in the ranks of the men.[68] Such individuals rejected the appeals to class made by the more class-conscious members of the labour movement.[69]

The oppositional nature of this proletarian public is evidenced by the efforts made to nationalize the health services of the country. Comments that the health services should be nationalized, or else socialized, were being made before the First World War[70] but it was during the inter-war period that more concerted, organized efforts were made. At the joint annual meeting of the Association of Approved Societies and the Association of Welsh Approved Societies in Cardiff in the summer of 1936, the chairman of the meeting, Evan Williams of Cardiff, opined that 'the co-ordination of the numerous agencies of medical service of every kind should be effected in the form of a State medical service'.[71]

That this 'State medical service' should be modelled on the medical aid societies of south Wales was the conclusion that some were coming to. The Political and Economic Planning (PEP) report on British health services of 1937 believed that the Llanelli and District Medical Service provided a 'comprehensive medical service which should be the model of any national system of medical services'.[72] Subsequently, the medical aid societies of south Wales were to have some influence on the shape of the NHS created in the post-war years. It has often been argued that Aneurin Bevan used his experiences of the Tredegar society, and his work on its hospitals committee, to aid him shape the NHS partly in their image. A rather Whiggish interpretation has been posited that considers the societies of south Wales to be an 'embryonic National Health Service'[73] but, as David Green has shown, these schemes did in some way serve partly to inspire the service created in the immediate post-war years. In a meeting with the Friendly Societies Medical Alliance and the South Wales and Monmouthshire Alliance of Medical Aid Societies during the planning stages of the NHS, Bevan told them: 'You have shown us the way and by your very efficiency you have brought about your own cessation.'[74]

Therefore the example of the medical aid societies, and the ascendancy of Aneurin Bevan to the heart of British political power, served significantly to influence the shape of the newly created NHS in 1948. The principle of paying for health care and attendance when well (through taxation in the case of the NHS) in readiness for periods of illness was as integral a part of the NHS as it had been for the societies. Bevan wrote that this was 'an act of collective goodwill and public enterprise and not a commodity privately bought and sold. It takes away a whole segment of private enterprise and transfers it to the field of public administration.'[75] This judgement of the NHS by Bevan could equally apply to the medical aid societies of south Wales. The working people of south Wales were, through their provision of medical services, recognizing the inadequacy of the system as it existed, were coming together as a public through the public use of their reason, and successfully created comprehensive medical services comparable to anything in Britain.

Conclusion

Habermas maintained that the public sphere he described was historically specific and was not to be transferred to other historical contexts. Nevertheless, his conception of the public sphere as the space within which private individuals could come together as a public to discuss and decide matters of importance, and its essential constitutive components of 'rational, critical debate' and popular participation, serves as a useful conceptual tool. It is evident that there existed in south Wales a proletarian public sphere founded on alternative values to the bourgeois, Liberal hegemony, although this is not to argue that these alternative values were not contested in the proletarian sphere. Nevertheless, with a strong tradition of self-sufficiency, the people of south Wales set about organizing their medical services on their own terms and in a way that addressed their particular needs. Despite government intervention and the opposition of the medical establishment, those people involved in the provision of medical services remained committed to the belief that health was not a private commodity to be bought and sold, but a civil right and a matter of social justice, and were relatively successful in putting many of their ideals into practice. 'The greatest good for the greatest number' was a lived ideal.

Notes

[1] I am grateful to Dr Paul O'Leary for reading an earlier version of this chapter and for making a number of comments and suggestions.

[2] Calhoun, C. (1992), 'Introduction: Habermas and the public sphere', in Calhoun, C. (ed.), *Habermas and the Public Sphere* (Cambridge, MA, MIT Press), pp. 1–2.

[3] Hesse, M. (1995), 'Habermas and the force of dialectical argument', *History of European Ideas*, 21, 3, 367–78.

[4] Hansen, M. (1993), 'Foreword', in Negt, O. and Kluge, A., *Public Sphere and Experience: Toward an Analysis of the Bourgeois and Proletarian Public Sphere* (London, University of Minnesota Press), p. xxvii.

[5] Outhwaite, W. (1994), *Habermas: A Critical Introduction* (Cambridge, Polity Press), p. 11.

[6] For criticisms of Habermas along these lines see Calhoun, 'Introduction'; Meehan, J. (ed.) (1995), *Feminists Read Habermas: Gendering the Subject of Discourse* (London, Routledge); Hesse, 'Habermas'; Cowans, J. (1999), 'Habermas and French history: the public sphere and the problem of political legitimacy', *French History*, 13, 2, 134–60; Brooke, J. L. (1998), 'Reason and passion in the public sphere: Habermas and the cultural historians', *Journal of Interdisciplinary History*, XXXIX, I, 43–67; I owe this last reference to Dr P. O'Leary.

[7] See Eagleton, T. (1984), *The Function of Criticism: From the Spectator to Post-Structuralism* (London, Verso), 35–6; Eley, G. (1990), 'Edward Thompson, social history and political culture: the making of a working-class public, 1780–1850', in Kaye, H. J. and McClelland, K. (eds), *E. P. Thompson: Critical Perspectives* (Cambridge, Polity Press), pp. 12–49; Negt and Kluge, *Public Sphere*; Tucker, K. H. (1996), *French Revolutionary Syndicalism and the Public Sphere* (Cambridge, Cambridge University Press); Breckenridge, K. (1998), ' "We must speak for ourselves": the rise and fall of a public sphere on the South African gold mines, 1920 to 1931', *Comparative Studies in Society and History* 40, 1, 71–108.

[8] See Green, D. G. (1985), *Working-Class Patients and the Medical Establishment* (Aldershot, Gower).

[9] Earwicker, R. (1981), 'Miners' medical services before the First World War: the south Wales coalfield', *Llafur*, 3, 2, 39–52; for comparable societies in America see Beito, D. T. (1997), 'The "lodge practice evil" reconsidered: medical health care through fraternal societies, 1900–1930', *Journal of Urban History*, 23, 5, 569–600.

[10] Foot, M. (1963), *Aneurin Bevan: A Biography*, vol. 1 (London, Readers Union), 63; Finch, H. (1972), *Memoirs of a Bedwellty MP* (Newport, Starling Press Ltd), pp. 33–5; Green, *Working-Class Patients*, p. 174.

[11] The population of the Tredegar Urban District was enumerated as 25,110 by the census of 1921.

[12] Gray-Jones, A. (1970), *A History of Ebbw Vale* (Risca, Ebbw Vale UDC), p. 245; the population of the Ebbw Vale Urban District was enumerated as 35,381 by the census of 1921; PEP (1937), *Report on the British Health Services* (London), p. 151.

[13] Earwicker, 'Miners' medical services', 41; Bedlinog Medical Committee minute book, 30 September 1924. Unemployed men were able to pay a reduced subscription of 3d per week; see also Tredegar Workingmen's Medical Aid Society, General Purposes Committee minutes, 13 July 1921. Some societies used the unemployed as collectors of subscriptions; see Maesteg Medical Fund Committee minutes, 28 January 1933.

[14] *Merthyr Express*, 25 January 1902.

[15] *Rhondda Leader*, 3 March 1900.

[16] Friendly and Benefit Building Societies' Commission, reports of the assistant commissioners, Ireland and Wales (1874), (C.-995), 12–13, 24–6.

[17] Arthur Horner characterized the relationship between the coalowners and the doctors as a 'sinister alliance'; Horner, A. (1960), *Incorrigible Rebel* (London, MacGibbon & Kee), p. 6.

[18] It was this tendency, argues Earwicker, that gave the south Wales clubs their distinctive character; 'Miners' medical services', 42.

[19] See for example *Report for 1912–13 on the Administration of the National Insurance Act*, part 1 (Health Insurance), Cd. 6907, 1913, xxxvi, part VI: National Health Insurance Commission (Wales), p. 480, where it was claimed that doctors 'chafed' under lay control.

[20] See for example *Llanelly Star*, 18 August 1934; 25 August 1934.

[21] *Merthyr Express*, 29 October 1904.

[22] *Rhondda Leader*, 17 October 1903.

[23] *Merthyr Express*, 24 September 1904.

[24] Ibid., 28 May 1904.

[25] Green, *Working-Class Patients*, p. 172.

[26] PEP, *Report on the British Health Services*, p. 151.

[27] For comments on the democratic nature of friendly society committees with obvious implications for the discussion of a proletarian public sphere here, see Green, David G. (1993), *Reinventing Civil Society: The Rediscovery of Welfare without Politics* (London, IEA Health and Welfare Unit), pp. 36–7.

[28] Earwicker, 'Miners' medical services', 41. Hilda Jennings, commenting on the deductions from miners' wages to pay for hospital treatment, a doctor, Welfare Fund, Sick Fund and Nursing Association, noted: 'The work of the various institutions is to a great extent governed by representative Committees of the miners, whose deliberations are marked by common-sense, shrewdness and a real desire for the common good'; Jennings, H. (1934), *Brynmawr: A Study of a Distressed Area* (London, Allenson), p. 71.

[29] These ballots were occasionally characterized by allegations of vote-rigging; *Caerphilly Journal*, 26 June 1920.

[30] *Merthyr Express*, 4 March 1911.

[31] Bedlinog Medical Committee minutes, 16 and 24 June 1922.

[32] *The Pioneer*, 18 October 1913.

[33] Bedlinog Medical Committee minutes, 1 October 1924.

[34] Maesteg Medical Fund Committee minutes, 17 January and 28 February 1931.

[35] As an example of this tendency Wil Edwards recounted the story of an elderly miner who, at an otherwise inconsequential trade union meeting in the late 1900s in Aberdare, stood up to address the meeting about the 'abnormal conditions' he was facing in his stall and advocated that at the very least there should be a minimum wage. In this way, the elderly miner coined a new phrase in the miners'

vocabulary and the 'minimum wage' was destined to be not only a phrase but also a phase in the miners' struggle against the coalowners. True or not, Edwards wanted this story to symbolize the democratic nature of trade unionism at that time and the way in which ordinary people could make their voices heard and influence great events; Edwards, W. J. (1956), *From the Valley I Came* (London, Angus and Robertson), p. 193.

[36] Pickering, P. A. (1986), 'Class without words: symbolic communication in the Chartist movement', *Past and Present*, 112, 144–62. In the context of the medical aid societies see for example *Aberdare Leader*, 19 April 1913.

[37] For examples see *Llanelly Star* and *Llanelly Mercury*, March 1934 to October 1935.

[38] Gwent Record Office, Tredegar Workmen's Medical Aid Society (D.3246.46).

[39] *Merthyr Express*, 25 June 1904.

[40] *The Pioneer*, 22 February 1913.

[41] *Llanelly Star*, 24 March 1934. See also *Llanelly Mercury*, 29 March 1934, which stated: 'The workmen have been bombarded with manifestoes and circulars.'

[42] *South Wales Gazette*, 24 September 1920.

[43] Ibid. For further information on Cox's attitude toward club practice in south Wales see Cox, A. (1952), *Among the Doctors* (London, C. Johnson), 172–6.

[44] *Merthyr Express*, 21 November 1903. These criticisms were dismissed by members of the committee, and the correspondent, E. Johnson, was accused of trying to secure a position for himself with the company; ibid., 5 December 1903; ibid., 26 December 1903; for other instances where the democratic nature of these club practices was called into doubt see ibid., 16 August 1902; the democratic nature of club practices controlled by employers was also criticized; ibid., 15 September 1906; 22 September 1906.

[45] However, the personal relationship and trust that developed between doctors and their patients also led workers to resist the changes advocated by a section of their colleagues. Similarly colliery officials and a certain section of the workforce were bought off by the 'gaffer intrigue' of doctors through bribes, free attendance and other subtle forms of manipulation; see for example *Western Mail*, 14 July 1900; *Rhondda Leader*, 1 February 1902; ibid., 29 March 1902; *The Lancet*, 28 October 1905, 1292–3.

[46] *Caerphilly Journal*, 21 August 1920.

[47] *Llanelly Mercury*, 23 August 1934.

[48] For examples of such language see *Merthyr Express*, 1 February 1902; ibid., 29 October 1904; *Rhondda Leader*, 23 September 1905.

[49] For examples see *Merthyr Express*, 11 January 1902; ibid., 25 January 1902; *Rhondda Leader*, 23 November 1907; *Aberdare Leader*, 29 March 1913; ibid., 19 April 1913.

[50] *Merthyr Express*, 25 January 1902.

[51] *Aberdare Leader*, 29 March 1913.

[52] *Merthyr Express*, 24 September 1904; time and time again, committee members and representatives of the workmen attempted to rouse the workmen to 'fight' for freedom and a better service: see also *Rhondda Socialist*, 23 November 1912 and 10 May 1913, the latter of which comments: 'We must insist on retaining the little freedom we now possess, and still keep fighting for more.'

[53] Ibid., 29 March 1934; see also 13 September 1934. At one point the workmen's committee accused the doctors of Hitlerism.

[54] Ibid., 20 September 1934.

[55] Ibid., 26 July 1934.

[56] *Llanelly Star*, 1 March 1934.

[57] Ibid., 13 October 1934.

[58] This supports John Pickstone's assertion that medical issues merge with the other activities of 'dominant' and 'subservient' groups and can be analysed as part of wider movements in local politics; see Pickstone, J. V. (1987), 'Medicine in industrial Britain: the uses of local studies', *Social History of Medicine*, 2, 2, 203.

[59] See, for example, the series of letters in the *Rhondda Leader* in the first few months of 1902 that urged the workers to 'awake' and 'arise', and to overthrow the older system of medical attendance; see especially *Rhondda Leader*, 18 January 1902.

[60] Eckley, S. and Bearcroft D. (1996) *Voices of Abertillery, Aberbeeg and Llanhilleth* (Strand, Gloucester, Chalford), p. 36.

[61] Foot suggests that the 'women worthies' were present on these committees when the employers still had a strong voice on them. The wives, sisters or aunts of company officials were present; Foot, *Aneurin Bevan*, pp. 49–50.

[62] On representation on the committees, see Tredegar Workingmen's Medical Aid Society Committee minutes, 26 April 1921 and Maesteg Medical Fund Committee minutes, 12 November 1932.

[63] *Neath Guardian*, 2 December 1938.

[64] As with disputes elsewhere the usual practice was for the workmen's committee to demand financial control, be refused by the doctors and then employ doctors who were willing to accept their terms. This type of struggle was repeated in many places in south Wales.

[65] *Caerphilly Journal*, 22 May 1920.

[66] See Smith, D. and Francis, H. (1980), *The Fed: A History of the South Wales Miners in the Twentieth Century* (London, Lawrence & Wishart), pp. 54–6; Williams, C. (1996), *Democratic Rhondda: Politics and Society, 1885–1951* (Cardiff, University of Wales Press), p. 208; Williams, C. (1998), *Capitalism, Community and Conflict: The South Wales Coalfield 1898–1947* (Cardiff, University of Wales Press), pp. 4–5.

[67] See Williams, R. (1980), 'Base and superstructure in Marxist cultural theory', in Williams, R., *Problems in Materialism and Culture* (London, Verso), pp. 31–49.

[68] Such divisions were not unlike religious schisms as competing factions disagreed over ideological and policy issues. For an example of a workman urging the men to stand together and not be divided see *Rhondda Leader*, 24 July 1909. One workman commented:

> Fellow-workmen, we are continually crying about the treatment meted out to us by the employers, but I think that the time is ripe for us to assert our rights among ourselves, and not form in parties and cliques, and sell ourselves for a mess of pottage, to be tools in the hands of people who have no sympathy whatever with us.

[69] Control of club practices seems to have been assumed by workers in other parts of Britain at an earlier date than was the case in south Wales; see Green, *Working-Class Patients*, pp. 70–87.

[70] A 'state medical service' integrating public and Poor Law health services had been advocated by the minority report of the Royal Commission on the Poor Laws

in 1909. In a Welsh context see for example *Merthyr Express*, 7 January 1911; *Caerphilly Journal*, 17 April 1920. In this latter instance a committee member of an Abertridwr scheme claimed 'that the time had come when the State should take over the entire control of the medical service of the country from top to bottom'. A similar call for the nationalization of the health services can be found in *Llanelly Star*, 25 August 1934.

[71] *Western Mail*, 4 July 1936.

[72] PEP, *Report on the British Health Services*, pp. 151–2.

[73] Foot, *Aneurin Bevan*, p. 63. Another biographer of Bevan, in stressing the experiences of the Tredegar society that aided Bevan to create the NHS, even went as far as to argue: 'These small Welsh mining towns were sometimes looked upon as the test-tubes of Socialism, where controlled experiments of a limited kind could be carried out under special conditions'; Brome, V. (1953), *Aneurin Bevan: A Biography* (London, Longmans), p. 49. See also Kinnock, N. (1998), 'Foreword', in Jones, G., *The Aneurin Bevan Inheritance: The Story of the Nevill Hall and District NHS Trust* (Abertillery, Old Bakehouse Publication), pp. v–vi.

[74] Quoted in Green, *Working-Class Patients*, p. 175.

[75] Ibid., p. 106.

6

Public Service and Private Ambitions: Nursing at the King Edward VII Hospital, Cardiff during the First World War

SARA BRADY

Introduction

Nurses working and training in Britain during the First World War had unique opportunities to fulfil private ambitions alongside their duties in public service. This was especially true for those living in geographically remoter areas and places with limited employment options for women. The war opened up employment for women generally and its impact was felt more strongly in a traditionally male-dominated and industrialized environment such as south Wales.[1] Nursing, however, offered a myriad of options – to become specialist nurses, for example, and to work abroad or in another institution. These skills and experiences could be carried over into their work after the war, and were not so easily pushed aside in peacetime, as was the work of many other women. The men returning from the battlefields, far from expecting them to move aside and back into the private sphere of the home, provided them with even more justification for professional acknowledgement. The two main pre-war occupations open to educated and mainly middle-class women in south Wales were nursing and teaching, although some dressmaking, shop and clerical work was also available. Nursing and teaching also provided some women with a stopgap between leaving school and marriage whilst learning skills considered useful for a housewife. Moreover, though the temporary employment of women in men's work during the war actively involved them in the war effort, nursing brought them closer still to the battlefront experience.

Nursing during the First World War was the closest most British women came to taking part in the action, as 'the experience of trench warfare . . . was a zone forbidden to women'.[2] Their experiences were unique because a 'nurse entered into a direct physical relationship with the wounded soldier'.[3] They were not only living in the public world of medicine, but also of war, and they were performing a public service as subordinates to doctors and military commanders. Their role was still an auxiliary one and 'masculine combat at the front was . . . more prestigious than feminine nursing outside the home or even at the front'.[4] This public service, however, allowed them to fulfil private ambitions more easily than ever before.

Nurses who wished to break away from their usual working environment, or who were not popular with senior members of staff and found their career paths blocked, were offered an escape route with the onset of war. The bargaining power of nurses at this time indicated a resistance to the element of social control in their recruitment, training, and working lives.[5] This suggests an upset in the balance of gender power, despite nursing for the military being considered a 'means of co-opting women for war service without threatening gender roles'.[6] This partial inversion of gender roles allowed nurses to utilize their public service to achieve their private ambitions. As Higonnet and Higonnet maintain, 'total war has acted as a clarifying moment, one that has revealed systems of gender in flux and thus highlighted their workings. Emergency conditions either alter or reinforce existing notions of gender, the nation, and the family.'[7]

Investigating the lives of nurses and probationers or trainees in a city such as Cardiff provides a 'provincial balance to the metropolitan experiences more usually described'.[8] Christopher Maggs's study, based around three Poor Law infirmaries in Leeds, Southampton and Portsmouth, and one voluntary hospital in Manchester, found that probationer records were helpful in revealing the 'appeal of the occupation in general', the way in which nurse probationers' education altered in response to the type of recruit who entered the profession, and 'the way in which nursing practice needed to take account of the characters of the nurses involved'.[9] Probationer records can also indicate social status, educational and employment history, and the geographical mobility of these women.

The Hospital

The King Edward VII Hospital originated as the Cardiff Dispensary that was set up in 1822 and moved to new premises in 1837, becoming the Glamorganshire and Monmouthshire Infirmary and Dispensary. It was known as the King Edward VII Hospital from 1911 to 1923, until it became the Cardiff Royal Infirmary. The Hospital formed the nucleus of the 3rd Western General Hospital during the war, and was the only base hospital in Wales. It was one of twenty-one general hospitals based on civilian hospitals which were set up to coordinate the treatment of sick and wounded military personnel.[10] Between 1914 and 1918 it relinquished a substantial amount of civilian resources to accommodate military needs, giving up 104 out of a total of 281 beds. The matron was Miss E. Montgomery Wilson, and ninety-one nurses were in her charge.[11] Staff from the hospital also worked in five local schools which had been converted to house the overflow of military patients, at Splott Road (surgical unit, 145 beds), Albany Road (surgical unit, 156 beds), and Lansdowne Road, Ninian Park and Howard Gardens (medical unit, 155 beds). A pupil teachers' centre was converted into a nurses' home accommodating seventy nurses.[12] Other hospitals in the Cardiff area also treated war casualties, such as the Welsh Metropolitan Military Hospital at Whitchurch (Cardiff City Mental Hospital).

The argument that hospitals can be seen as microcosms of the society in which they develop can be applied to the King Edward VII, a financially comfortable, philanthropic, paternalistic and ambitious institution, that acted as a reflection on Cardiff as a whole.[13] Colonel E. M. Bruce Vaughan was the major influence behind fund-raising for the hospital from about 1900, and he was credited with turning around its fortunes.[14] By 1917, donations to the hospital to commemorate the war had reached £40,000, half the amount required, and appeals were made for ward and bed subsidies: 'what better tribute to the memory of a soldier who has given his life for his country and his God could there be than one from which their fellow-men will in their need benefit "for all time".[15] In addition, Anthony House, a privately donated property, was opened on 1 August 1917 as a preliminary training school for probationer nurses.[16] Newly sponsored wards were also opened, including a maternity flat and a new orthopaedic department in 1917. Many working men donated via the 'Penny-a-week' scheme – for example from the Senghennydd and Abertridwr collieries – and local businessmen and colliery owners contributed heavily, thereby exercising a paternalist concern. Finally, the ambition of the hospital was evident in the debate raging at the time over the opening of a medical school in Cardiff, centred around the King Edward VII. Bruce Vaughan was heavily involved with the campaign for a Welsh medical school and felt there was a need for a 'School of Research in Wales, which England, Scotland and Ireland have had for centuries, and poor little Wales must do without . . . unless her Members of Parliament will insist there should be no further delay'.[17] Finance for the project was to come partly from private funds, most notably from Sir William James Thomas, one of the major benefactors of the hospital. Thomas had offered £10,000 to build a new physiological laboratory in 1912, increasing this amount to £30,000 if the Treasury gave a grant for a new Welsh school of medicine to be started.[18]

The hospital annual reports in the early period of the war gave the impression of a financially secure institution, but this changed as expenditure exceeded income in later years. Though the financial effect of the conflict was not immediately apparent, members of the various fund-raising committees published appeals for money that exploited the new circumstances. In the 1914 annual report, for example, they tapped into popular support for the war by encouraging public sympathy for nurses helping with the war effort: 'Again the scores of Nurses, splendidly trained women, who are tending the sick and wounded in France and Belgium and at home – as well as our Civilian sick and invalids – *were educated and trained in our Hospital.*'[19]

By 1915, the financial strain was beginning to show. 'The increase in cost per occupied bed is due to the enhanced prices of practically everything, and to the expense borne by the Hospital on account of the military patients', argued the annual report for that year.[20] Military use of the new orthopaedic ward and the electrical pavilion built in 1905 was proudly advertised:

we have treated no fewer than 122 officers, non-commissioned officers, and men and pensioners, with a total number of 650 treatments in this part of the month . . . And such is the provision for treatment with regard to space and equipment that we shall be able to treat another 100 pensioners (orthopaedic cases) a week if the War Office will find us the personnel.[21]

But at the same time, the hospital Board of Management was anxious about the cost of accepting military patients as this seriously affected the treatments and number of beds available for civilian use. Fund-raising activities increased, and concern was expressed in the annual reports that civilians would become weary of donating to the hospital whilst receiving a diminished service. However, despite this tension with the military role, hospital staff were inevitably working simultaneously in the public spheres of medicine, the hospital, and the war. And the disruption this caused enabled many to alter their lives in ways that would not have been possible before. The remainder of this chapter explores how nurses at the King Edward VII could combine public service with their own private ambitions.

Voluntary Aid Detachments

Voluntary Aid Detachments (VADs) were organized into local groups of volunteer amateur nurses after the development of the 1909 'Scheme for the Organisation of Voluntary Aid in England and Wales' to prepare auxiliaries for the professional military nursing of the Queen Alexandra's Imperial Military Nursing Service (QAIMNS) and the Territorial Force Nursing Service.[22] Groups were organized by the Red Cross and the Order of St John, and the VADs attended residential camps as well as short training courses at local hospitals.[23] In 1914, there were around 80,000 VADs in Great Britain, and by 1918 this had increased to around 120,000.[24]

The King Edward VII Hospital did not appear to be keen to take on voluntary nurses on an *ad hoc* basis and turned down several requests for individual basic training. In 1914, there had been some confusion when a 'misunderstanding [was] abroad with reference to the lack of facilities given to Members of the St John Ambulance

Association, the British Red Cross Society, and the Royal Army Medical Corps (RAMC) for training at the Hospital'.[25] It was, however, reported in 1915 that

> satisfactory arrangements were made, through the kind co-operation of the Matron, to afford the members of the British Red Cross Society and the St. John Ambulance Association opportunities to gain practical experience in the routine work of a Hospital. The experience consists of a three weeks' course of training in the Ward and various departments.[26]

In total, 113 VAD members of the British Red Cross Society and sixty-five members of the St John Ambulance Association trained at the hospital for military service.[27]

In 1915 thirteen special probationers also trained there prior to undertaking military work. A special meeting of the Nursing Committee was held to discuss a letter from the British Red Cross Society asking the Board of Management to 'consider the possibility of allowing carefully selected members of the Women's Voluntary Aid Detachments to be admitted to the Wards, Kitchens, Laundries and even Store Rooms and Linen Room of the Hospital'.[28] This gives an idea of the type of work they were expected to do and the domestic nature of much of it.

Whilst the King Edward VII Hospital played host to a number of VADs during this period of staff shortages and increased patient load, they were generally considered to be the equivalent of domestic helps, and were unlikely to receive the training required for professional nursing. Much of the friction between VADs and trained nurses was caused by what was considered the former's challenge to the professionalism of the latter, especially because of the disparity in their civilian social status. VADs were mostly from the upper classes, whilst many nurses were from middle- and lower-class backgrounds. Notable VADs from the locality included Miss Olwyn Lloyd George, who went to France in 1915 to work at a base hospital in Boulogne, and Miss Margaret Chrichton-Neate, Commandant of VAD 24 Glamorgan from August 1914, who worked as a masseuse for the 3rd Western General Hospital.[29]

Despite the growth of nursing, there was still a shortage of staff at the outbreak of the war, leading to the influx of volunteers. This meant that VADs as well as probationer nurses often found themselves in positions of greater responsibility and urgency than would normally have been the case. Patients could not easily distinguish between untrained and professional staff, which caused much resentment in those who were fully qualified.

Probationers

The School of Nursing, established early in 1888, was the first centre for paramedical education to open at the King Edward VII Hospital.[30] The 155 probationer nurses, who began training between 1911 and 1918 at the King Edward VII Hospital, were likely to have had some experience of nursing during the war. The Nurse Training Record books were used to record detailed personal information about the probationers and provide much of the source material referred to below. The data recorded included personal details such as nationality, age, address and occupation of the head of household, education, previous work experience, and religion. The Hospital Nursing Committee minute books provide additional material of a more general nature relating to both probationer and qualified nursing staff and the contemporary issues surrounding their work.

The records kept for the probationers were in most cases complete, at least as far as personal details are concerned. Details such as age, home address, education, previous employment and father's or husband's (if widowed) occupation, were indicators of social status. They also demonstrated examples of unusual instances or non-standard candidates, which can indicate a flexibility in recruitment. Despite the low drop-out rate, there was towards the end of the war a slight increase in the number who gave up their training before completion; five left in 1914 and seven in 1918, with a fall to less than five per annum in the intervening years. Possible hypotheses for this are that some left to get married to their partners returning from the front, or that they lost interest in nursing as a profession after the excitement of the war years. Maggs suggests in his work on hospital recruitment between 1881 and 1921 that the failure of many nurses to complete their training was possibly a general trait of women's employment at the time.[31]

The occupation of the father or husband contributes to an indication of the social status of probationers. The most common occupations of heads of household were as follows: agriculture (19), retired (7), building (6), teaching (5), religious (3), professionals (surgeon, veterinary surgeon, coroner, lawyer, 3 civil engineers, 2 bank managers, architect, surveyor, and accountant), and trades (2 grocers, 2 bootmakers, draper, and smith). Overall, occupations indicated a broad mix of income and status. A minority of the probationers came from backgrounds of a higher status, with head of households such as gentleman farmer and surgeon, but the majority were of a lower social status than these.

The probationer intake from Wales for 1911 to 1918 was 120, the majority from south Wales, including twenty-four from Cardiff. There were only two from Aberystwyth representing mid-Wales. Seventeen came from England (five of these had been born in south Wales), sixteen were from Ireland, one from Scotland, and one from Australia. Eight of the Irish probationers were from Miltown Malbay in Co. Clare, which points to a possible recruitment link with this area of Ireland. The records therefore indicate a wide variety of geographical origins for this limited sample of probationers, suggestive of the hospital's status and reputation, and of advertisements being placed outside the local area.

The age limits on recruits, generally between twenty and thirty, meant that there was a period of time for potential nurses between school and hospital training that had to be usefully filled. These women helped at home or worked in other occupations, depending on their families' financial circumstances. The King Edward VII files state ages of new recruits from 1911 to 1918 as between nineteen and thirty-nine. The majority were in their early twenties. Four began training at the age of nineteen. The eldest was thirty-nine years old, and there were eight others in their thirties. Maggs states that during the late nineteenth century, the age range for nurse training was between twenty-five and thirty-five years.[32] The *Welsh Outlook* described a far more rigid recruitment process:

> An intending nurse usually begins her training at the age of 23 or 25 at one of the large hospitals, and at 20 or 21 in a children's or special hospital. Thus there are half-a-dozen years, more or less, to be passed after leaving school before she enters a hospital.[33]

However, the growth in hospital care needs meant more nurses and so a subsequent relaxing of these criteria was inevitable.

Individuals were considered for their all-round appropriateness for training, and age did not appear to be a major barrier to recruitment. Under the conditions of war, it would appear that the power to bend the conventions was conferred upon the Nursing Committee and in particular the matron.

The previous employment of the probationers recruited between 1911 and 1918 shows that fifty had nursing experience working at various institutions around Great Britain, and one in France. Fever, isolation, cottage, military and ophthalmic hospitals, a maternity home, and sanatoriums were represented, such as the Welsh Metropolitan Hospital, Whitchurch; the Pembroke Dock Military Hospital; Laurels Red Cross Hospital, Neath; St John's Hospital, Barry Island; and the Red Cross Hospital, Maesteg. This cross-section of previous hospital experiences indicates that some probationers were taking up training places with prior knowledge of what would be expected of them. Only some of the institutions were of similar or greater stature than the King Edward VII, such as St Bartholomew's in London. The majority of them were smaller and less prestigious, but they were useful stepping-stones into the nursing profession. If these were formal probationerships, then it was possible that a contract with the previous hospital may have been prematurely ended to take up the new post.

Social Status

Examination of the social backgrounds of these women enables closer scrutiny of the connections between their status and power, and that of the hospital. Disparities in social status continued to divide women during the war years, in contrast to the experience of many soldiers in the trenches brought together by their experiences.[34] The differences between those women of high or middling social status were sustained by the divisions between probationers and VADs, and engendered competitive ideals that were not synonymous with the traditional concept of nursing as selfless work.

The *Welsh Outlook* reported that 'numbers of Welsh women have applied for a month's training in nursing with the view to proceeding to the front at the end of the month to work in the field hospitals'.[35] The article commented on how ridiculous this was, arguing that three years was the very least amount of training required. It recommended hospital training as the 'royal road'. Underlying this support for nurses in training for the usual minimum of three years, and criticism of volunteers looking for a short cut into nursing, was a solidarity of social status with them. The article expressed the importance that the voluntary hospital placed on nurses and their position of social respectability, on which untrained VADs had no right to impose their perceived superiority.

The war provided opportunities for trained nurses to be posted overseas, to have some choice in where they worked and to take advantage of being a highly sought-after resource. They argued that they had worked hard for their status, only for it to be usurped in some cases by VADs of higher civilian social status. Whilst the soldiers were supposedly bridging the class divide by their wartime experiences, many women were just discovering how wide the gaps were, and fighting to preserve their own status. Nursing may have brought women of different classes into closer physical proximity, but social cohesion was not necessarily the result. It was the first time for many that they were enabled to travel away from home and into the wider world, having even less opportunity than men of their respective class. The war gave them the perfect chance to escape the restrictions of their normal existence and experiences. The nurses at the King Edward VII were involved in this exercise of personal fulfilment and private ambition through travelling abroad and working in military units as well as treating casualties at Cardiff.

Like the women's suffrage movement as a whole, the Cardiff and District Women's Suffrage Society – the largest and wealthiest branch of the National Union of Women's Suffrage Societies (NUWSS) in south Wales – was actively engaged in supporting hospitals during the war.[36] It had close links with the Scottish Women's Hospitals (SWH) organization, whose founder, Dr Elsie Inglis, was an active member of the NUWSS. The SWH was recruiting staff from around Britain, who consisted mainly of women, including doctors, nurses and VADs.[37] A contingent from the SWH visited Cardiff in April 1915, where Dr Inglis gave a talk at City Hall to raise funds for the organization and to equip a Welsh Hospital for Serbia. Amongst the supporters at the meeting were Mrs Lloyd George, and Mrs R. Lewis, president of the South

Wales and Monmouthshire Federation of Women's Suffrage
Societies.[38] Subsequently a Welsh Committee set up an appeal for
the Welsh Hospitals Unit for Serbia, which was started in 1915
under the auspices of the Newport and Cardiff branches of the
NUWSS.[39] It helped fund the SWH Valjevo Unit, headed by Dr
Alice Hutchinson, which served in Serbia from May to November
1915.[40] A group of forty SWH nurses, under the command of Dr
Hutchison, sailed from Cardiff in 1915, as reported in the *Western
Mail*, which described the visual impact of the nurses in their grey
uniforms as they walked through the town.[41]

The staff of the Scottish Women's Hospitals organization
included women from all over Britain:

> The National Union (NUWSS) . . . and more particularly the Scottish
> Federation, may well feel proud . . . to tell that the Scotchwomen who
> wear the tartan are of the same dogged staying breed as the men who
> wear it in the trenches. The English and Irish and Welsh members
> scattered amongst the Staff are proud to wear it too, as the soldier
> wears the decoration of another nation out of compliment . . .[42]

The SWH's links with Wales could have provided an important
advertisement for voluntary nursing. A nurse from Bargoed became
a local heroine after working in voluntary service in Serbia with the
Scottish nursing contingent and being captured and taken to
Austria. When she arrived back home there was a reception committee at Aberbargoed railway station and a procession marched
through the local villages behind the nurse in an open carriage,
surrounded by an armed escort.[43] The absence of any similar
organization to the SWH in Wales was possibly due to lack of a
national medical school and a network of Welsh women doctors.
The apparent eagerness of Welsh medical staff, including nurses, to
associate themselves with the SWH and the Welsh Overseas
Hospitals indicates that Celtic and national identity were important to many in their employment choices.

Training and Professional Status

By the time war broke out in 1914, nursing had been in a trans-
itional state for about thirty years. The greater popularity of

hospital treatment was evident from the growth in medical institutions funded by the Poor Law authorities as well as from the expansion of charitable voluntary hospitals. Therefore, the demand for nurses grew. Nursing having become a respectable occupation, like teaching, mainly for middle-class women, and for those who saw it as a vocation and a career, the work became more sophisticated. It no longer consisted of purely domestic-type duties because medical and surgical techniques changed and more in-depth knowledge and specialized care were required. Institutions had begun to evolve their own training programmes to suit the needs of their medical specialists and the patients they accepted.

Voluntary hospitals were independent in their training and terms and conditions, but Poor Law authorities were able to organize their services more uniformly via their more cohesive management.[44] Despite previous reluctance to pass a registration Bill, the government's position changed at the outbreak of war. With so many VADs flooding into the nursing service, and public sympathy and support for nurses, politicians saw some reasons for accepting change.[45] The probationers of the King Edward VII Hospital were recruited into an evolving profession as, in 1919, the Nurse Registration Act and the General Nursing Council came into being, and three years' training including examinations to be passed became standard.

An awareness of status differentials within nursing was shown by G. Arbour Stephens MD in *The Hospitals of Wales*, published in 1912. Despite considering hospitals to be a superior training environment for nurses, he valued the Poor Law hospitals more highly than the voluntary hospitals. Arbour Stephens considered that the 'Nurses trained at the voluntary hospitals of Cardiff and Swansea pride themselves upon the superiority of their certificates', but claimed that they were not so well adapted for private work and were too specialized.[46] Too keen to do 'elaborate surgery', they became 'infected with the spirit of excitement . . . of daring operations'.[47] He argued for the standardization of nursing examinations and training for the 'good of the Nation', and wrote in nationalistic terms arguing for the university to work more widely throughout Wales, for all to benefit and for training to be more widely available for potential staff. His argument that the University of Wales was too elitist demonstrated an awareness of the discrepancies of status within health care work and training, as well as between institutions. To achieve a higher social and work status, better opportunities for nurses were to be found by working at large voluntary hospitals. Nurses in less prestigious institutions fitted the more traditional model of the nurse, working vocationally in a caring environment without much opportunity for self-development. Those with ambitions to enhance their status, or at least to maintain it, and to gain personal satisfaction from their post, could achieve more if they already came from a more advantaged position in life. The war, however, made it easier for others to push at the social boundaries. During the nineteenth century, '[n]ursing offered a career structure, a rare opportunity for women, but its potential was restricted by the low status accorded to basic care and the stance taken by doctors and some of the reformers themselves'.[48] The experience of nurses during the war years changed this considerably.

Wartime probationers came to nurse training from a variety of educational backgrounds that included state elementary, intermediate and county schools, commercial and charitable institutions, and home tuition. The 1870 Elementary Education Act had provided educational opportunities for the poorer working class and lower middle class in self-contained elementary schools, with a compulsory age limit of thirteen imposed in 1876.[49] Subjects taught at this level, such as reading, writing and arithmetic, could be supplemented with some scientific teaching.[50] Education beyond this level developed through higher-grade schools and scholarships to the intermediate or secondary schools.[51] W. Gareth Evans argues that the 1889 Welsh Intermediate and Technical Education Act counteracted to some extent the gender bias in education. He stated that '[t]eacher training had provided a limited form of higher education for Welsh women', although the 'domestic ideology fed to working-class girls . . . was a notable feature'. By the early twentieth century, however, 'there [was] a greater awareness of the dangers of gender stereotyping'.[52] The amount of scientific teaching offered to girls continued to be deficient.

Despite nursing being more biased towards housekeeping than medicine, probationers had to take examinations in scientific subjects such as dispensing, physiology, anatomy, gynaecology and surgical nursing. In an article on women training to be doctors between 1890 and 1939, Carol Dyhouse discussed a similar problem of how women frequently needed private tuition in scientific subjects to gain university entrance. They had often only been taught some basic biology or botany.[53] The King Edward VII was regarded as a modern institution that kept up with scientific and medical advances. The nurses were expected to work in the new electrical pavilion and do theatre work, for example, which required a good level of education and training. Seven of the probationers took and passed the six-month training course in massage. One also passed examinations in X-ray and medical electricity. All of them had to make up the time lost from their training at the end of their course. These specialist skills became sought after post-war for convalescing military patients, but they were something that VADs would not have experienced.

Wartime shortages meant that there were fewer staff to give training of any kind, and probationers had to take on more responsibility. In 1916 there was a serious shortage of staff in the operating theatre, and a third-year probationer was asked to stand in as a theatre nurse. As Maggs states, the war was important for nursing as it highlighted the '[l]ack of numbers to care for this increased patient-load' as well as the different emphasis required in a military hospital.[54] This completely altered the dimensions of nursing from its central civilian health care role.

Over 200 nurses from the hospital had served at the Front by 1917.[55] The 'Need for Nurses' was expressed in the *Welsh Outlook*: 'There is always a great demand for nurses and especially for Welsh speaking nurses; that demand at the present moment is intensified as a result of the war.'[56] There were new opportunities for nurses from the hospital to participate in war-related work. Nurses could earn higher wages and move to other parts of the country or abroad with relative ease during the war. Even probationers could gain valuable experience training with new medical techniques and treatments, and take on more responsibility. The remaining staff and probationers at the King Edward VII were increasingly valued as the war progressed, especially as advertisements for new staff received only one or two replies, if any. The secretary of the Nursing Committee reported that 'so many nurses were leaving the Hospital after obtaining their certificates in consequence of the inducements offered by Military Service, the nurses at present on the Staff of the Hospital not caring for the work, and no applications having been received in response to advertisements'.[57] The matron and other senior staff were increasingly weighed down with other responsibilities and their concern was expressed in the Nursing Committee minutes. In October 1914, the matron was already reporting difficulties in arranging for adequate training for probationers because of the number of beds in use by the military authorities.[58]

To cope with recruitment and training problems, the hospital administrators had to offer competitive wages in line with those offered by hospitals around the country; indeed, the records show that they contacted other institutions regarding salary scales. On 23 March 1915 it was reported that the Nursing Committee had considered the question of salaries after receiving information from other hospitals. It came to the conclusion that owing to the '[g]rave and growing shortage of Sisters and Staff Nurses . . . every possible inducement should be offered to retain staff and attract applicants'.[59] This could benefit the nursing staff more than the hospital, as the former could increase their labour value and career prospects, whilst the latter had to accommodate them as best it could to retain their services. The hierarchical structure of the hospital was therefore threatened in so far as it had to increase its flexibility to meet the demands of nursing staff. The Nursing Committee had also decided to increase the wages of one sister and three staff nurses who belonged to the Territorial Service, but had not been mobilized as their services were required at the hospital.[60] Despite the curtailment of their ambition to undertake military work, they could be partially satisfied with a pay increase. It would not have been impossible for them to leave for another post even after this decision by the hospital authorities.

Of the 155 records in the sample of probationers, forty-eight indicated post-training nursing employment. The majority became staff nurses (thirty-six), with two becoming sisters. Four did private nursing, and two were school nurses. Ten did some form of military work directly, including five who became Territorials, three who went to the Welsh Hospital, Netley, and two who worked at the Whitchurch Military Hospital. One, a surgeon's daughter, left to study medicine.

A considerable contribution to staff shortages at the King Edward VII Hospital was caused by the Welsh Hospital. It was established in October 1914 in the grounds of the Royal Victoria Military Hospital at Netley, Southampton, and recruited heavily from south Wales, and Cardiff in particular. Nursing staff had come from the King

Edward VII, as well as the dispenser and some medical officers. The majority of the staff had some Welsh connection.

Casualties arrived at Netley direct from the incoming troopships or by train to its own railway station. One such casualty was the poet Wilfred Owen. He spent ten days at the Welsh Hospital in June 1917 suffering from shell-shock and wrote to his mother, 'It is pleasant to be among the Welsh – doctors, sisters, orderlies. And nurses.'[61] The temporary hospital building provided an unusual working environment for the nursing staff as it was a timber and corrugated-iron structure which could be dismantled to be transported abroad at short notice.[62] An exhibition, held in aid of funds for the Hospital from 13 to 18 December 1915 in Cardiff, stated in its brochure that the building was originally intended to be placed in France, but was built at Netley 'in deference to the wishes of the Army Authorities'.[63] It was 'the first voluntary Hospital to be offered to, and accepted by, the War Office'.[64] The sense of national pride felt for the Welsh Hospital was evident in a 1915 article: 'our neighbours are drawn from all parts of the UK, but they all agree to envying the Welsh Hospital.'[65] This was possibly a light-hearted dig at the nearby Irish Hospital which was built shortly after the Welsh.

As already discussed, trained nurses moving to military postings such as at Netley could earn more money and broaden their career experience. A sister from the King Edward VII served at Netley, on leave of absence, for six months, from October 1914. When she requested further leave for six months to continue her work there, her request was supported by Lt.-Col. Alfred Sheen, the commanding officer/senior surgeon who was also from the King Edward VII Hospital. Despite this, the Nursing Committee reluctantly withheld permission owing to a 'grave shortage of Senior Nurses at the Hospital'.[66] In 1916, the sister was eventually given leave to serve with the Welsh Overseas Hospital, but without the possibility of having her position at the King Edward VII Hospital retained.[67] Although she would have no job to return to when the war ended, the sister was willing to accept the consequences of fulfilling her private ambitions. Three months prior to its opening, a Cardiff woman who had recently received an appointment in Liverpool as the matron of a tuberculosis hospital wired offering her services as matron of the Welsh Hospital, which was supposedly to go to the front.[68]

Conclusion

Nursing during the First World War consisted of many strata, as can be seen on a primary level with the differences between VADs and qualified and probationer staff. These distinct groups could also be identified with specific social statuses – the lower and middle status with trained nursing staff, and the higher status with VADs. The friction between them helped to fuel the ongoing debates regarding nurse training and registration. Whilst the need for proper training and registration was revealed in its full importance because of the distinction required from VADs, the latter also helped to raise the profile of nursing and hospital care in the eyes of many patients who would normally have used private help at home. Women who nursed may have been viewed as a homogeneous group by some patients, but the differences between them were acute to the nursing staff themselves. Public service was an element of the motivation for the majority, but private ambitions were also a driving force, whether for a career, travel or any of the other openings that the war offered.

Examining the personal training records of probationer nurses at the King Edward VII Hospital indicates that the majority were from middle-class backgrounds. Information such as their geographical origins, father's occupation, education and age provided a useful resource to ascertain more exactly their social status. They had to be educated well enough to cope with the training and examinations. Generally aged between twenty and thirty, they had the social and educational advantages to enable them to advance their careers and to travel away from home. Previous occupations give an indication of the experiences of recruits prior to becoming probationers, and the many who had already done some nursing provide evidence of consistency in ambition. Post-training employment, where recorded, shows continuation of a career in nursing in most cases. Whilst it is impossible to say whether this would have been the case if the war had not taken place, the decision to undertake military work by the newly qualified, as well as those already working at the hospital, was a proactive one, as they remained very much in demand for civilian work.

The hospital, the city of Cardiff, the support of the NUWSS, and connections with other military hospitals at home and abroad, such as the Scottish Women's Hospitals and the Welsh Hospital, offered nurses many new and varied job opportunities. The wage increases received by qualified staff enabled them to experience better financial security and the flexibility to change jobs. New developments in medical treatments, and diverse patient types, also offered fresh experiences, specialization and job satisfaction. The hospital included nursing staff in its investment for the future, by actively encouraging diversification and specialization, such as in massage and electrical treatments. Not all contemporaries agreed that nursing specialization was beneficial to patients. However, the popularity of the hospital as a local institution was evident in its ability to retain reasonable financial health during the war. It managed to build on its already well-established means of support and to retain wealthy benefactors. The increase in the treatment of soldiers and officers benefited the hospital by encouraging a wider variety of patients to attend.

The nursing staff and probationers appeared keen to engage in their nursing careers and the war presented them with many opportunities. For those already enrolled or working, it built on the experiences they already had. For new recruits, perhaps encouraged by the war effort to enrol in nursing, they began in an advantageous position. Staff were required in growing numbers, broader experiences were available, higher wages were being paid on qualification, and promotion could progress more rapidly. Promotion was not necessarily easier, though, as the hospital records show that posts were left empty rather than being filled by the wrong candidate. Despite increased benefits that enabled staff to satisfy their personal ambitions, they remained in positions of public responsibility within a hospital whose management rigorously maintained its professionalism throughout the war. In this way, the hospital administration refused to upset social and gender roles. Away from the confines of the hospital it was possible to invert these roles, through travelling and working abroad, dealing with patients direct from the front, living in hazardous conditions, choosing where to work and applying for posts that offered the most in fulfilling private ambitions. All this was achievable in wartime whilst still undertaking public service and outwardly remaining within the prescribed roles for nurses and other women.

Notes

[1] Beddoe, Deirdre, 'Munitionettes, maids and mams: women in Wales, 1914–1939', in John, Angela V. (ed.) (1991), *Our Mothers' Land: Chapters in Welsh Women's History 1830–1939* (Cardiff, University of Wales Press), pp. 188–209.

[2] Tylee, Claire M. (1990), *The Great War and Women's Consciousness: Images of Militarism and Womanhood in Women's Writings, 1914–64* (Basingstoke, Macmillan), p. 8.

[3] Summers, Anne (1988), *Angels and Citizens: British Women as Military Nurses 1854–1914* (London, Routledge & Kegan Paul), p. 273.

[4] Higonnet, M. R. and Higonnet, P. L. R. (1987), 'The double helix', in Higonnet, M. R. et al. (eds), *Behind the Lines: Gender and the Two World Wars* (New Haven, Yale University Press), p. 35.

[5] Granshaw, L. and Porter, R. (eds) (1989), *The Hospital in History* (London, Routledge), p. 3.

[6] Summers, *Angels and Citizens*, p. 278.

[7] Higonnet and Higonnet, 'The double helix', 5.

[8] Maggs, Christopher, 'Nurse recruitment to four provincial hospitals 1881–1921', in Davies, Celia (ed.) (1986), *Rewriting Nursing History* (London, Croom Helm), p. 19.

[9] Ibid.

[10] Richards, John (ed.) (1994), *Wales on the Western Front* (Cardiff, University of Wales Press), p. 217.

[11] *The Hospital*, LVI, 12 September 1914, 656–7.

[12] *The Hospital*, LVII, 14 November 1914, 151–2.

[13] Granshaw and Porter, *The Hospital in History*, p. 4.

[14] Evans, Neil, '"The First Charity in Wales": Cardiff Infirmary and south Wales society, 1837–1914', *Welsh History Review*, 9 (1978–9), 319–46, p. 319.

[15] *King Edward VII's Hospital, Cardiff, Annual Report, 1917*, pp. 29–30.

[16] *Annual Report, 1917*, p. 25.

[17] *Annual Report, 1915*, p. 39.

[18] Ibid., pp. 41–50.

[19] *Annual Report, 1914*, p. 33.

[20] *Annual Report, 1915*, p. 24.

[21] *Annual Report, 1917*, pp. 29–30.

[22] Summers, *Angels and Citizens*, p. 274.

[23] Ibid.

[24] Abel-Smith, Brian (1960), *A History of the Nursing Profession* (London, Heinemann), p. 85.

[25] *Annual Report, 1914*, p. 26.

[26] *Annual Report, 1915*, p. 28.

[27] Ibid., p. 118.

[28] Nursing Committee minute books 1909–18, 19 February 1915.

[29] Jones, Robin (1989), *History of the Red Cross in Monmouthshire (Gwent) 1910–1918* (Pontypool, Raven Press), and (1919), *The Honourable Women of the War and The Women's (War) Who's Who* (Bournemouth, W. Mate and Sons).

[30] Aldis, Arnold S. (1984), *Cardiff Royal Infirmary 1883–1983* (Cardiff, University of Wales Press), p. 38.

[31] Maggs, 'Nurse recruitment', p. 38.

[32] Ibid., 20.

[33] *Welsh Outlook*, 1 (November 1914), 456.
[34] Higonnet and Higonnet, 'The double helix', 44.
[35] *Welsh Outlook*, 1 (November 1914), 456.
[36] Cook, Kay and Evans, Neil, ' "The petty antics of the bell-ringing boisterous band"? The women's suffrage movement in Wales, 1890–1918', in John, *Our Mothers' Land*, p. 171.
[37] Leneman, Leah (1998), *Elsie Inglis* (Edinburgh, NMS Publishing Ltd).
[38] Jones, *The Red Cross in Monmouthshire*, p. 89.
[39] Beddoe, Deirdre (2002), *Out of the Shadows: A History of Women in Twentieth-Century Wales* (Cardiff, University of Wales Press), p. 64.
[40] Ibid.
[41] *Western Mail*, 21 April 1915.
[42] Quoted from 'Common cause', in McLaren, Eva Shaw (ed.) (1919), *A History of the Scottish Women's Hospitals* (London, Hodder & Stoughton), p. 21.
[43] *Cardiff Times*, 4 and 11 March 1916.
[44] Nursing Committee minute books 1909–1918, 19 February 1915, 1323.
[45] Abel-Smith, *History of the Nursing Profession*, pp. 82–3.
[46] Arbour Stephens, G., MD (Lond.) (1912), *The Hospitals of Wales* (Swansea, Lewis Evans), p. 35.
[47] Ibid.
[48] Cherry, Steven (1996), *Medical Services and the Hospitals 1860–1939* (Cambridge, Cambridge University Press), p. 34.
[49] Lawson, John and Silver, Harold (1973), *A Social History of Education in England* (London, Methuen & Co. Ltd), pp. 318–22.
[50] Ibid., p. 330.
[51] Ibid., pp. 338–9.
[52] Evan, W. Gareth (1990), *Education and Female Emancipation: The Welsh Experience, 1847–1914* (Cardiff, University of Wales Press), pp. 257–8.
[53] Dyhouse, Carol (1998), 'Driving ambitions: women in pursuit of a medical education, 1890–1939', *Women's History Review*, 7, 3, 326.
[54] Maggs, 'Nurse recruitment', p. 23.
[55] *Annual Report, 1917*, pp. 29–30.
[56] *Welsh Outlook*, 1 (November 1914).
[57] Nursing Committee minute books 1909–18, 8 August 1916.
[58] Ibid., 6 October 1914.
[59] Ibid., 23 March 1915.
[60] Ibid., 2 March 1915.
[61] Hoare, Philip (2001), *Spike Island: The Memory of a Military Hospital*, (London, Fourth Estate), p. 253, quoted from Owen, *Collected Letters*, p. 470.
[62] *The Hospital*, 24 October 1914, 95, quoted in Richardson, Harriet (ed.) (1998), *English Hospitals 1660–1948: A Survey of their Architecture and Design* (Swindon, Royal Commission on the Historical Monuments of England).
[63] *The Welsh Hospital, Netley*, 1915, brochure.
[64] Ibid.
[65] *Cardiff Times*, 7 August 1915, 3.
[66] Nursing Committee minute books 1909–1918, 23 March 1915.
[67] Ibid., 1 May 1916.
[68] *Cardiff Times*, 22 August 1914.

7

'Fit to Work': Representing Rehabilitation on the South Wales Coalfield during the Second World War

ANNE BORSAY

Introduction

For the documentary movement in inter-war Britain, film opened up a new 'public sphere'[1] by enabling informed debate in the mass media and not just through the 'face-to-face communication' of Habermas's Enlightenment ideal.[2] The argument in this chapter revolves around a five-minute sequence called 'Fit to work' which explains how the Caerphilly District Miners' Hospital and the Talygarn Rehabilitation Centre at Pontyclun in the Vale of Glamorgan treated industrial injuries on the south Wales coalfield during the Second World War. Four main themes are examined: the nature of the documentary film; the policy context of local rehabilitation services; the interface between nation, citizenship and medicine; and the implications of this relationship for constructions of class, gender and disability. Finally, the conclusion will assess how far the documentarists succeeded in creating an enlarged public sphere.

The Documentary Film

'Fit to work', directed by Donald Alexander (1913–93) and produced by Paul Rotha (1907–84), was released towards the end of

1944 as part of a bi-monthly magazine called *Worker and War-Front*. This series, introduced two years before under the auspices of the Ministry of Information, was designed for non-theatrical rather than cinema distribution and viewed by workers in the war industries at factory and social venues.[3] Technological innovation and the expansion of television have turned the documentary tradition from which this kind of information film emerged into a multifaceted medium that is no longer reduced to the original 'expository' mode where the visual was deployed to underline the authority of the lone narrator. Until recently, however, the academic debate was dominated by the feature genres whose fictional content aligned itself more easily with the literary culture that propagated film studies. Only in the 1990s did the postmodernist challenge to reason and truth rekindle interest in the realism of the documentary and its commitment to purvey objective knowledge.[4] Yet by the 1930s, 'the factual film was already a highly sophisticated structure, a great deal of interpretation being implicit in the original selection and editing, and frequently including a mixture of bits and pieces taken at other places and other times as well as the use of "justifiable" reconstruction.'[5]

Film-makers recognized the subjectivity that these procedures involved. John Grierson – founding father of the documentary movement who inspired its activities first from the Empire Marketing Board and then from the GPO Film Unit – described the medium as 'the creative treatment of reality'. Paul Rotha – producer of 'Fit to work' – agreed that 'creative art' was brought into 'observation'.[6] Critics like Brian Winston have pointed to 'the obvious contradiction in this formulation'. 'The supposition', he says, 'that any "actuality" is left after "creative treatment" can now be seen as being at best naive and at worst a mark of duplicity.'[7] There are two problems with this accusation. First, objective knowledge being in tatters, the 'ideal of the pure documentary uncontaminated by the subjective vagaries of representation' has to be abandoned for 'a new definition of authenticity . . . that eschews . . . the transparency of film and replaces this with a performative exchange between subjects, filmmakers/apparatus and spectators'.[8] Second, the documentary movement was open in its commitment to the 'bending to social purpose of actuality'.[9] Its vision of the post-war world was a left-wing one – born of an abhorrence of inter-war poverty and deprivation, and depicted in films like *The*

Nation's Health (1935) and *Housing Problems* (1935). Both film-makers associated with 'Fit to work' shared this political mindset. In 1935, whilst still a Cambridge undergraduate, Alexander made a short silent film called *Rhondda* with the Socialist Films Council.[10] And Rotha, renowned for his radicalism, was later accused of using the *Worker and War-Front* series to plug 'hard-line pro-paganda' of Soviet descent which advocated 'a great central planning authority of experts'.[11] Such allegations of an 'open conspiracy' are exaggerated.[12] Politicians and civil servants were busy with other aspects of the Ministry of Information's wide-ranging brief and allowed the documentarists a high degree of 'creative freedom'.[13] Churchill – though happy to eulogize the 'broad sunlit uplands' that would accompany peace[14] – avoided concrete commitments which might detract from the war effort by provoking controversy. The Labour Party, on the other hand, held the principal domestic portfolios in the coalition government after 1940[15] and the public debate about a future welfare state was invigorated by publication of the Beveridge Report in 1942.[16] It was this space that the documentary filled.

The Policy Context

In the policy context of the Second World War, rehabilitation exemplified the reforming agenda of the documentary movement, making the innovative accident service at the Caerphilly hospital and the Talygarn centre an appealing vignette. Rehabilitation acquired prominence after 1939 in the main due to the labour needs of the wartime economy. Its definition was broad. For the 1945 *Hospital Survey* of South Wales and Monmouthshire, rehabilitation was:

> part (but only a part) of a process of restoring, as far as possible and in the shortest possible time, the full mental and physical, and therefore working, capacity of a patient whose mental and physical health has been impaired because of sickness or accident.[17]

The concept was historically rooted in the inter-war alliance between preventive medicine and the clinical speciality of ortho-paedics. Public health, argued the chief medical officer of health in

1926, embraced not just the avoidance but also 'the removal of the occasion of disease and physical inefficiency, combined with the husbanding of the physical resources of the individual'.[18] Orthopaedics applied this thinking to its two principal patient groups, 'crippled' children and fracture cases. But though doctors increasingly represented physical disability as a preventable or curable condition, the number of 'crippled' children was declining as the incidence of rickets and tuberculosis fell. Therefore, the management of fracture cases became the engine for change, joining maternal mortality and morbidity as one of the pre-eminent inter-war health issues.[19]

Orthopaedics had greatly enhanced its professional reputation during the First World War by promoting an expertise in the treatment of locomotor injuries which were often fractures caused by bullets and shrapnel. In the depressed post-war economy, however, suffering from a surplus rather than a deficit of labour, rapid return to work offered little inducement to develop effective rehabilitation services.[20] Consequently, a study by the British Medical Association in 1935 showed that more than half the fractures treated each year were maladministered, that 37 per cent of patients in one sample were disabled for the rest of their lives, and that, critically, three-quarters of all cases were still handled primarily at home.[21] The official response to such shocking findings included a committee to consider 'the rehabilitation of persons injured by accidents'. Its final report, published just before war broke out, confirmed that the lack of specialist care for fracture cases produced a 'gravely defective' system of treatment. Furthermore, there were warnings that these limitations would be aggravated by the incidence and severity of war injuries.[22]

By the summer of 1939, the Emergency Medical Service had come into being and requisitioned more than a half of all hospital accommodation for casualties of the conflict.[23] The effect was not immediately to rectify previous bed shortages, and although there were twenty-four orthopaedic centres in preparation by the beginning of 1940, anxiety about continuing underprovision led to the establishment of an Inter-Departmental Conference on the Rehabilitation of Persons Injured through Enemy Action. The conference was disturbed to find both civilian and military hospitals failing to refer patients for whom they were neither staffed nor equipped, and teams of advisers were appointed to 'worry' hospitals into

complying with specialist referral. The realization that enemy
bombing caused fewer major orthopaedic casualties than
estimated allayed some of this concern. However, the extension of
the Emergency Medical Service to civil defence and industrial
workers aggravated the pressure, and in March 1941 fractures were
still regarded as 'badly treated'.[24]

The response to this deficiency was soon to be revolutionized by
the manpower shortage. First, the orthopaedic centres were rapidly
joined by 'several hundred' fracture departments and clinics with
less specialist briefs. Second, an 'Interim Scheme' for engaging
disabled people in the war industries was introduced which linked
hospitals, and hence medical advice, to employment exchanges and
training centres. This initiative was consolidated from late 1942 in
a third phase after the government accepted the Report of the
Inter-Departmental Committee on the Rehabilitation and Resettle-
ment of Disabled Persons. The committee, under the chairmanship
of George Tomlinson MP (1890–1952), 'recommended an extension of rehabilitation methods to all areas of the country, and to
other patients besides those with fractures – medical and surgical
patients, the blind, and people suffering from tuberculosis, neur-
osis and other illnesses'. The Ministry of Health reacted by undertaking a rehabilitation survey of the hospital services and inviting
selected institutions to appoint rehabilitation officers. Equipment,
clothing and supplies for physiotherapy and occupational therapy
had been distributed to over 400 hospitals by the end of 1943, and
others had been provided with prefabricated gymnasia or with
grants and licences to adapt their premises. Training courses for
doctors and physiotherapists were also set up to address the
shortage of qualified staff. The scheme was dramatic in its effects,
almost doubling the number of hospitals using rehabilitation
methods within twelve months.[25]

Rehabilitation on the South Wales Coalfield

Rehabilitation on the south Wales coalfield occurred within this
national policy context, building on existing medical institutions in
an effort to frame a coordinated strategy. Medical aid societies had
sprung up in the Valleys from the 1870s, bringing together major
local employers and their workforces to organize free treatment

and entitlement to sick pay. These societies were to the forefront in developing voluntary hospitals.[26] In Caerphilly, the mining community initially contributed to the Cardiff Royal Infirmary, and this support was commemorated in the naming of wards after local collieries. By the end of the First World War, however, Caerphilly lodges, working through the East Glamorgan District of the South Wales Miners' Federation, had arranged for a weekly levy to be subtracted from wages to finance an infirmary.[27] Most of the £42,000 required to purchase the former house of a master sinker and convert it into the Caerphilly and District Miners' Hospital came from this source, with only £3,250 – less than 10 per cent – being donated by local colliery companies.[28]

Workmen's contributions were also the major source of revenue after the premises opened, supplying over 90 per cent of income in 1924 – the first full year in which the hospital was operational.[29] The number of beds had risen from twenty-three to eighty-four, plus an outpatient department by 1930, when the facilities were extended beyond industrial injuries to treat miners' wives and children.[30] Moreover, in 1939 the Ministry of Health was paying almost £1,800 for fifty additional emergency beds. That payment aside, the income profile of the hospital was remarkably stable, especially given the deep inter-war Depression in south Wales which undercut voluntary funding.[31] Donations and subscriptions trebled to £255 between 1924 and 1939, and diversified to include not just personal gifts but also the proceeds of sporting events, musical concerts and dances, and special picture shows. In addition, the hospital organized a fête and gala. None the less, at the outbreak of the Second World War the hospital was still obtaining virtually 90 per cent of its total ordinary income from the contributions of the local workforce.[32]

The increase in beds expanded the flow of patients through the hospital; in 1924 there were 205 admissions, in 1939 there were 780. Yet despite this growth, the clinical profile was relatively unchanged; in 1924, 40.5 per cent of patients were 'chronic surgical cases' and 59.5 per cent were accidents or 'other emergencies for operation'; in 1939, 44.3 per cent of patients were surgical cases 'from the waiting list' and 55.7 per cent were accidents and emergencies.[33] Recorded clinical outcomes during the period improved. Not only did the death rate fall from 6.6 to 2.8 per cent, but the proportion discharged as 'cured' rose from 82.4 to 94.5 per cent. The hospital was staffed by general practitioners, supported by regular visits from consultants.[34] In the absence of clinical records, we cannot reconstruct the therapeutic regimes which they used to achieve these results. However, the annual report, which in 1924 referred only to massage, was in 1939 also listing 'radiant heat', 'galvanism', 'faradism' and 'ultra violet ray light'. The implication is that patients were being exposed to a varied range of treatments which led the *Hospital Survey* to describe the Caerphilly regime as 'progressive'.[35]

The Talygarn Rehabilitation Centre was likewise regarded as an advanced facility. Talygarn was a nineteenth-century mansion built by the scholar ironmaster, G. T. Clark (1809–98): the surgeon, civil engineer and public health inspector who later managed the Dowlais ironworks in Merthyr Tydfil, served local boards for education, health and poor relief, and authored both a study of medieval military architecture and a county history of Glamorgan.[36] In 1922, Clark's grandson sold the house and grounds to the South Wales District Committee of the Miners' Welfare Commission.[37] The commission had been established by the Industry Act of 1920, on the recommendation of the Sankey Commission which investigated the nationalization of the coalfields in the trail of their collectivist control during the First World War.[38] Its job was to administer the Miners' Welfare Fund, created under the same legislation by levying a charge on every ton of coal raised. Its terms of reference, as outlined in section 20 of the Act, were to apply these moneys 'for such purposes connected with the social well-being, recreation and conditions of living of workers in or about coal mines and with mining education and research'.[39] Between 1937 and 1945, the levy generated £900,000 for such uses in south Wales alone and the total amount spent in the region exceeded £2,000,000.[40] Though the commission was perhaps best known for halls and institutes, pithead baths and canteens, £80,000 had been allocated to hospital projects by the end of the Second World War.[41]

Convalescence was also a concern. And it was with this in view that the South Wales District Committee paid £16,500 for Talygarn and spent a further £10,000 on conversion; a home was to be provided in which 105 miners could 'recuperate during a two weeks' stay under ideal conditions'.[42] In 1938, no fewer than 2,678 residents passed through Talygarn, and 'from the inception of the

Home in October, 1923, to December, 1939, a total of 41,222 patients . . . [were] admitted'.[43] However, the Home Committee had long realized that Talygarn 'did not effectively serve the purpose for which it was intended, partly because of its location, the unsuitability of the building due to its heavy upkeep costs, and the weather conditions prevailing in South Wales generally'. Consequently, when the parent Miners' Welfare Commission sought to buy the home in 1943 and turn it into a rehabilitation centre for injured miners, the negotiations were successful. A convalescent hotel was acquired in Bournemouth where, it was argued, 'the climate will more than compensate for . . . [the] little discomfort' of a longer journey.[44] Meanwhile Talygarn entered a new era of its life. Wards became rooms for occupational therapy, remedial games and physiotherapy; the concert hall became a gymnasium; a new block was built 'to house surgical examination facilities, a plaster room, craft and work rooms, and an X-ray department'; and specialists in orthopaedics and rehabilitation joined the staff. Finally, the length of stay for the seventy patients now accommodated was determined by the treatment programme which their injuries necessitated.[45]

Like the Caerphilly District Miners' Hospital, Talygarn was a cog in the government's rehabilitation machine, its new regime recognized by the *Hospital Survey* as a 'great success' with 'a limited range of traumatic disabilities among miners and some other workers'.[46] In the rehabilitation sequence of *Worker and War-Front*, the narrator told a story about these two model institutions. In the opening scene, a woman emerged from her home holding a small child as the emergency siren sounded at the mine. The movement from private to public sphere drew the audience into an industrial landscape of pitheads and slag heaps, and began a journey which was both geographical and narrative.[47] A haulage man had fractured an arm when trapped under a tram. Skilled first aid by his workmates and a careful transfer from the site of the accident to the ambulance room at the surface reduced the risk of further damage. The victim was then transported to the Caerphilly hospital – one of seven specialist fracture centres on the coalfield set up by the Emergency Medical Service – where his arm was set by a dedicated orthopaedic surgeon and placed in a plaster cast. Once able to travel, he was moved to Talygarn for a rehabilitation programme which rendered him 'Fit to Work'. This travelogue thus

tracked the miner from rescue underground via the hospital to
Talygarn,[48] and articulated the progress from injury to rehabilitation in a way which conformed to the classic problem-solving
dynamic of the documentary.[49] Moreover, though short and sparse,
its representations of nation, citizenship and medicine, class,
gender and disability, threw into sharp relief a cluster of socio-
political values and relations that were pivotal not only to wartime
policies but also to the post-war welfare state.

Nation

Wales personified the nation as an 'imagined political community',[50] possessed of diverse, competing and evolving identities.[51] In
'Fit to work', the urban/rural divide was played out most
evocatively. Indeed, so pervasive was the shadow of industrialization
that the location was intuitable even before the opening
commentary revealed that 'something serious has happened at this
colliery in south Wales'. The reason was the filmic legacy of the
coalfield. Some contributions were feature films like *The Citadel*
(1938) and *How Green Was My Valley* (1941), based on novels by A.
J. Cronin and Richard Llewellyn respectively. But public perceptions
of Wales were likewise influenced by the documentary footage
which had turned the coalfield into a 'photogenic and dramatic'
source for fiction film-makers.[52] As well as making the Rhondda
film, Donald Alexander directed *Eastern Valley* (1937), which dealt
with a cooperative food scheme in Gwent. John Eldridge – another
leading figure of the documentary movement – was responsible for
Wales: Green Mountain, Black Mountain (1942), with a narrative
by Dylan Thomas desperately trying to reconcile rurality and
industry. And the polymathic Humphrey Jennings – painter, poet,
literary scholar and co-founder of the social survey Mass
Observation, as well as film-maker[53] – transposed a Nazi massacre
in Czechoslovakia to west Wales when he made *Silent Village* (1943)
with the help of the South Wales Miners' Federation.[54]

Though the rural dichotomy feeding these images of raw
urbanism was derived from the documentarists' English identity,
with its late Victorian ambivalence towards industrialization,
Welsh culture also had an arcadian ideal of similar vintage which
was likewise promoted by 'a loose coalition of middle-class

radicals'. Via organizations such as the interdenominational Welsh School of Social Service, this group sought to transmit the values of rural peasants and artisans to the proletariat of the Valleys. For them, Welshness was 'an attitude of mind' to be inculcated by education and religion; and it was envisaged that the 'national sentiment' which ensued would permit the resolution of industrial conflict and social injustice through the regulation of market capitalism.[55] This political mentality was not unequivocally shared by the south Wales miners. Yet a rural aesthetic of health was endorsed. Therefore, just as the Sully Tuberculosis Hospital – built in the mid-1930s for the Welsh National Memorial Association – was designed to maximize the sunlight and fresh air of its coastal site on the Vale of Glamorgan,[56] so the Talygarn Centre was seen to capitalize on its rural environment.

In August 1946, *The Miner* – the official journal of the South Wales Miners' Federation – dedicated a special issue to Talygarn. Among the illustrations was a photograph of two patients sawing wood: an image symbolizing the oneness of man and nature, and

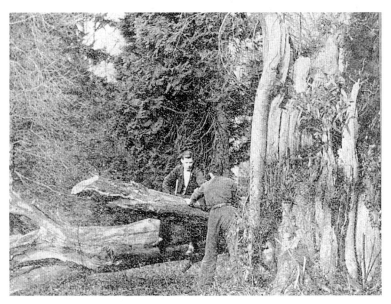

Figure 7.1 Talygarn Rehabilitation Centre: one of the exercises (*The Miner*, August 1946; courtesy of the South Wales Miners' Library, University of Wales Swansea).

the healing properties of the two when acting in harmony
(Figure 7.1).[57] Furthermore, the centre's remote location, and the
natural beauty of the gardens and grounds, received lavish praise.
It was:

> situated on an elevated position in the midst of choice and rare
> specimens of valuable and ornamental timbers of all shapes, hues and
> classes . . . in the varying lights and shades of our weather and the
> multi-coloured shades and tints caught by the light rays, indescribable
> beauty – fragile as gossamers, perfect in beauty and resplendent in
> majesty – abounds as if mocking at the intruder, who is so limited when
> he could be so profound.[58]

This effusive description testified to how contested Welsh identities
were. A state of mind for the inter-war nationalist movement,
rurality was also harnessed by trade unionists to symbolize
recovery from industrial accidents in a publicly financed institution. Common to both, however, was the aspiration for economic
and social change.

Citizenship

The rehabilitation programme conducted at Talygarn blazed a trail
for the 'social corporatism' that was to characterize the welfare
state and, therefore, it afforded the documentarists an excellent
arena in which to map out a national culture based on a reformed
relationship between the citizen and the state.[59] The concept of
citizenship that they favoured was derived from the idealist
philosophies of Kant (1724–1804) and Hegel (1770–1831), im-
ported from Germany in the second half of the nineteenth century
and influential for thinkers like T. H. Green (1836–82) and F. H.
Bradley (1846–1924). This school of thought did not deny the
importance of working-class agency. On the contrary, schemes of
self-help and mutual aid were welcomed for their cohesive properties. However, unrestrained individualism was berated for failing to hold society together and a bureaucratic model of the state
was championed in which the expert reigned supreme. Within this
political framework, the responsibility of the documentary film
was to educate the citizen, informing him (*sic*) of how – in Sidney

Webb's words – he might best fill 'his humble function in the great social machine'.[60]

All these themes were played through in 'Fit to work'. First, the film recognized the importance of working-class participation. Not only did the commentary reveal that the Caerphilly hospital was 'built and run by the miners themselves' and that trade unionists were actively involved in the management of Talygarn, but colliers were also exhorted to learn the first aid skills needed to help each other when accidents occurred underground. Second, the creative intervention of the state was emphasized in setting up fracture centres across the coalfield and coordinating a rational system of transfer to specialist facilities. And, finally, professional expertise was rarefied.[61] Consequently, the patient was constructed as a passive recipient of advice who had to be cajoled into persisting with long-term rehabilitation rather than accepting a short-sighted financial package. It was

> no longer a question of fighting for compensation but rather fighting to get a man fit again by giving him the best of specialist treatment. For today the emphasis is not on whether the injured man will have enough to live on when disabled but on how soon and how completely the accident service can fit him to carry on his old job . . .

Donald Alexander's longer drama documentary on rehabilitation, made as early as 1941 and cheerfully entitled *Life Begins Again*, was similarly positioned, representing fracture patients discharged from hospital as helpless victims, idle and demoralized without the spur of professional advice and direction.

Medicine

Since medical expertise underpinned rehabilitation, the dominant message of 'Fit to work' was the ability of doctors to cure industrial injuries if only given the chance. Much stress was placed on rapid access to expert care, symbolized by a uniformed procession of trolleys at the Caerphilly hospital; the white coat – first put on in the laboratories of the mid-nineteenth century – was 'the ultimate symbol of the marriage of science and clinical medicine'.[62] This therapeutic optimism was rooted in the emergence of scientific medicine as, from the later eighteenth century, disease became disconnected from 'the experience of the sufferer and relocated . . . in a system of thought about the human body based on the findings of pathological anatomy'.[63] But within the profession itself, orthopaedics was a poor relation. Managing shock did involve the use of technology – blood transfusion, plus the radiant heat, galvanism, faradism and ultraviolet ray light, all of which were listed in the Caerphilly hospital's annual report for 1939. However, long-term rehabilitation centred on the coordination of paramedical practitioners, and although orthopaedic surgeons tried to elevate plaster casts into icons of modernity, the bone-setting that was their principal craft fell short of the scientific paradigm.[64] Therefore, when 'Fit to work' revealed that four out of five patients returned to full employment underground, it was the multidisciplinary regime at Talygarn that was most celebrated.

The marginality of orthopaedics to mainstream medicine encouraged an allegiance with the trade union movement which since the later 1930s had endorsed specialist treatment and jointly campaigned for the reform of workmen's compensation.[65] The effect of this partnership was to set in motion a powerful process of objectification. Not only were 'forms of knowledge originally embedded within everyday life . . . separated and subjected to specialist development',[66] but this separation was promoted by working-class leaders as well as medical practitioners. In south Wales, scientific rehabilitation was vigorously sold through the pages of *The Miner*. Writing in October 1944 for the very first issue, W. J. Saddler claimed that '[t]he medical profession accepts the responsibility of a cure; they affirm that there is no need for the fracture to permanently cripple the workman'. Indeed, they had 'almost performed miracles'. As well as casting aspersions on 'the local medical practitioner . . . unskilled in the proper treatment of fracture cases', Saddler attacked the traditional bonds of family and community which had sustained injured miners. Remembering his own time in the pits, he criticized the 'very crude improvised stretchers' that were used to take men home 'over very long distances on the shoulders of their workmates'. Once there, they were

> left . . . to be washed by willing but unskilled hands of the neighbours.
> The fracture had to come right of itself, when placed between two
> splints for days and weeks until some sort of union had taken place,

[and the patient was abandoned] to cure himself . . . [by] the toning-up of his injured muscles.[67]

The August 1946 issue of *The Miner* likewise denigrated family and community care by stressing the 'primitive conditions . . . in old Welsh mining cottages', and the inadequacy of nursing patients 'by the fireside' and treating shock with hot-water bottles.[68] Such privileging of medical knowledge was visible and audible throughout 'Fit to work', there being neither camera shots from patient angles nor interruptions in the official narrative for patient voices.[69] Yet the image of stretcher-bearers conveying an injured man into the hands of caring relatives and neighbours was a powerful statement of local solidarities which the objectified doctor–patient relationship, conducted within institutional environments, was unable to replicate. Medicine sequestrated the accident experience.[70]

Class

The professional expertise championed by the documentary film not only obscured the recipient of rehabilitation services; acting in conjunction with the underlying concept of citizenship, it also encouraged stereotypical notions of class, gender and disability. Despite making working people worthy of serious filmic attention,[71] the documentarists approached the deprived communities of inter-war Britain like strangers from afar, much as Victorian philanthropists entered the slums or Victorian imperialists penetrated darkest Africa.[72] The visual and textual content of 'Fit to work' exemplified this outlook. The first image of mother and child was set against a valley backdrop which gradually closed in and hence constructed the viewer as a visitor from outside.[73] Both the problem of industrial injury and the solution of rehabilitation were then presented by the narrator through middle-class eyes, and the message was delivered in a didactic way which testified to the gulf between the classes.[74] Above all, Talygarn was said to have been 'conceived by the former owner of the great Dowlais steelworks', G. T. Clark. The mansion, of course, was; but the Miners' Welfare Commission had purchased it from his grandson, thus invalidating the hint of industrial paternalism.

Trade unionist representations of Talygarn challenged this patronizing view of the working class. True, there were traces of deference in the elaborate description of 'The Home', produced in a 1930s publicity brochure and later repeated:

> The costly panelling and carving in the Reading, Writing and Billiard Room, the Reception Hall and the Main Corridor, represent many fine examples by Biraghi, effected in 1895; the work for the most part by this well-known Italian Artist being in the Venetian Style, depicting various Allegorical Subjects, Heraldic Devices, Cupid and Caryatide Figures, Scrolls and Arabesques featuring Labour, Art, etc. There are also some very massive and finely carved Carrara Marble Mantelpieces.[75]

However, if this account – so alien to the poverty of the Valleys – evidenced a sycophantic attempt to civilize the lower orders by exposing them to an elite culture, it was undercut by a counter-vailing sense of social solidarity. For residents, the 'tonic of comradeship' was vital to the experience of recovery. '[A]lthough none of the patients might be known to you', wrote one in October

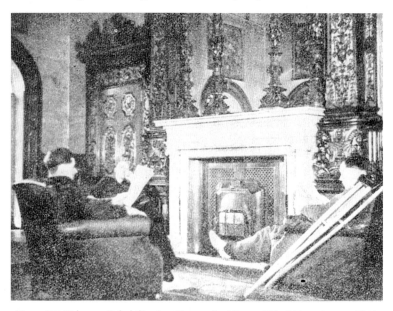

Figure 7.2 Talygarn Rehabilitation Centre: the Library (*The Miner*, August 1946; courtesy of the South Wales Miners' Library, University of Wales Swansea).

1946, 'you very soon realise the wonderful spirit of friendship . . . that prevails and endures towards you . . . everyone is delighted to assist his colleagues along, and you will make friends you can never forget.'[76] In turn, this mutual support, and the institutional context within which it occurred, was seen as a shot across the bows of the class structure. Therefore, the patient who relayed the interests of fellow inmates to the matron and treatment staff was called the 'captain': a military rank not easily accessible to a miner. Furthermore, the special issue of *The Miner* included a large photograph, showing three men with their newspapers around the fire (Figure 7.2).[77] This was a metaphor of invasion. Social class was temporarily subverted. Working people were making themselves at home in a gesture of social equality.

Gender

Whereas trade unionist imagery relieved the class-bound perspective of the documentary movement, it offered no respite from the rigidities of gender and disability. The madonna figure of the first 'Fit to work' sequence, which fixed the viewer as an outsider, also peddled an idealized picture of the wife and mother which bore little resemblance to the drudgery of women's lives either on the coalfield itself[78] or in the factories where the film was shown. Throughout the Second World War, government policy towards the employment of women was similarly contradictory, the Ministry of Health lauding their domestic role and the Ministry of Labour their economic role.[79] By late 1942 gender relations at work were tense, as female morale plummeted and male resentment at women's employment was expressed through harassment, non-cooperation and discrimination by the trade unions. The feature film, *Millions Like Us*, released at the height of this unrest in 1943, was conciliatory, attempting 'to win over that part of the female audience which was unsure of . . . war work by suggesting that the pleasures of love were the inevitable accompaniment and reward'. Conventional feminine virtues – 'obedience, industriousness, uxoriousness' – were approved; conventional masculine virtues – 'physical strength', 'authority', 'leadership' – were sanctioned.[80]

In the context of the mining industry, the 'physical strength' of the labouring man was a particularly powerful stereotype which

reinforced women's domestic role. Though 'Fit to work' devoted
little space to the romanticized masculinity that Beatrix Campbell
has called 'male narcissism', other documentaries like *Industrial
Britain* (1933) and *Coalface* (1935) depicted the working male in
heroic terms as brave and ennobled by physical labour; and where
his body was allowed to eclipse a worship of the machine, it was
pictured close-up as broad and muscular. Conditions underground,
with men extracting coal semi-naked, fuelled this imagery.[81] But
the stripped male bodies were also vulnerable, as the recitation of
accident and death rates underlined.[82] And with industrial injury
the threat to the idealized body materialized. Neither the sanitized
reconstruction of the accident scene at Caerphilly,[83] nor the shots
of the rehabilitation regime at Talygarn, conveyed much sense of
the suffering involved in mending broken bodies. Indeed, even *The
Miner* made light of the issue by stressing that supervisors and
instructors took '[g]reat care . . . to ensure that no patient exerts
himself beyond his . . . capacity, by so arranging the exercise and
games as not to be too exacting on the physique of the injured
man.'[84] In practice, however, it seems likely that men were pushed
to the outer limits of endurance within a closed masculine world
where peer group pressures intensified the valiant drive towards
normality.

Disability

Rehabilitation's mission to reinstate a compliance with able-bodied
norms, irrespective of the physical pain or mental anguish
involved,[85] undermined the citizenship of disabled people. Therefore, rather than accepting impairment as a legitimate human
condition and recognizing that total recovery was not always an
appropriate goal, 'Fit to work' communicated that the injured
miner could once more be made a 'useful and normal citizen'. *The
Miner* adopted a comparable language to the documentarists in an
article on the Disabled Persons (Employment) Act of 1944.
Sheltered workshops were embraced enthusiastically for the
severely disabled person 'who could not be expected, either for the
rest of . . . [his] li[fe] or for a long time, to stand up to the hurly-
burly of industrial life in full competition with non-disabled
workers'. This was the way to 're-establish for him normal family

life, normal employment and normal recreation, and reinstate him in the privileges and duties of citizenship'. This was the way to ensure that '[a] disabled man, despite his disability, . . . [was] an asset and not a burden'.[86]

The linkage of citizenship to productivity and normality initially appears uncontentious. After all, unemployed Rhondda miners talking in Ralph Bond and Ruby Grierson's film, *Today We Live* (1937), welcomed help from the National Council for Social Service but observed that it was no substitute for proper work.[87] Moreover, disabled people, likewise keen to find jobs, were enthusiastic about the new opportunities that opened up as a consequence of war, and over 300,000 either obtained work or training after the government introduced its special recruitment scheme in 1941. Official information films like *Back to Normal* (1945) pictured disabled workers expressing optimism about their post-war prospects:

> A lot of people . . . think that if you've only one arm they've got to get you an easy job like a clerk or a lift attendant. At first I thought they were right. But if you've been an engineer – what's wrong with the same job? I find I can manage pretty well and it's a simple matter for a government training centre to give you the correct tools.

Without the crisis of a wartime economy, however, positive attitudes to the employment of disabled people faded, as Gerald Turner – a young man with cerebral palsy searching for a job in the late 1940s – discovered: 'I went to the Labour Exchange and they just used to throw me out and say there wasn't any work for somebody like me. They didn't think I was any use to anyone.'[88]

The reasons for this reversal were discernible even during the war. The news media eulogized the achievements of disabled people, praising men like 'Blind John', a farmer from Northumberland who carried on milking the cows and delivering to customers despite his visual impairment.[89] However, such lives were presented as heroic, individual victories over adversity. Consequently, there was no understanding of disability as a societal construction manufactured by material and cultural environments;[90] as 'the disadvantage or restriction of activity caused by a contemporary social organization which takes no or little account of people who have physical impairments and thus excludes them from the

mainstream of social activities'.[91] This 'social model', which came
to prominence from the 1970s, has recently been accused of ignoring both the physical and the psychological suffering of impairment, and the multiple identities which arise from class, race and
gender.[92] None the less, its focus on the structure of society does
explicate the pairing of work and normality by flagging up a commitment to maximum 'efficiency, productivity and material progress'.[93] War briefly extended the parameters of economic activity
for disabled people, but the old logic was preserved in the concept
of citizenship advanced by the documentary movement and
enshrined in the Beveridge Report. Therefore, even the welfare
state failed to come to terms with the able-bodied unemployment
which had so obsessed the Victorian Poor Law. Labour-market
participation remained the priority. Claimants with insufficient
National Insurance contributions continued to be restricted to
stigmatizing means-tested assistance.[94] And disabled people who
were not fit to work found that post-war policies neglected their
needs in health and housing, education and social services,
transport and environmental design.[95] Citizenship came with
employment conditions attached.

Conclusion

The grounding of citizenship in economic rather than political
status institutionalized the 'abnormality' of those whom the
rehabilitation machine could not repair. But to what extent did
these images – and the portrayals of nation, gender and class –
shape perceptions within a bigger public sphere? The documentarists were confident that cultural artefacts were capable of
forming as well as reflecting opinion;[96] like other elements in the
inter-war intelligentsia, they assumed that the encounters with
actuality which they constructed had the power to transform the
thoughts and actions of audiences not previously exposed to such
debates.[97] Historians have tended to concentrate on the feature film
and play down the importance of the 1,400 short documentaries
with which the Ministry of Information was associated during the
Second World War.[98] Nicholas Pronay, for instance, has insisted:
'As far as the war effort was concerned, the country could have
dispensed with the whole lot without an iota of difference. The

real propaganda *war*', he concludes, 'was carried out in the commercial cinemas and by the newsreels, not in any significant way by the documentary.'[99] More recently, however, Richard Barsam has put the opposite case, arguing that 'the documentary film movement did influence social thinking, . . . and contribute significantly to the nation's efforts in World War II'.[100] So how do we assess these competing viewpoints?

The weekly audience that watched non-theatrical productions – 360,000 at its peak in 1943/4 – was small in comparison with weekly cinema attendance of 24 million.[101] Nevertheless, over a third of all shows each week were given to large groups in factory canteens, and approximately 2,000 sites were visited once a month with some multiple viewings for different shifts.[102] The reception of documentaries screened in these settings is difficult to gauge. Though cinema audiences and exhibitors complained about the quantity and quality of information films,[103] *Worker and War-Front* was a novel mix of information and entertainment,[104] designed 'to link the home front with the combat front'[105] and to nurture social integration by sharing the experiences of different employment communities or spelling out the implications of a routine job.[106] 'Fit to work' was therefore sandwiched between an episode on how rockets were loaded into Hawker Typhoon fighter planes, and an act by the popular comedian, Tommy Handley. Paul Rotha believed that the formula was 'very popular, very success-ful';[107] and the Ministry of Information staff who distributed films were enthusiastic too, taking heart from the voluntary way in which bookings were made.[108] But were these views justified?

The mission of public education which *Worker and War-Front* shared had the potential to engage audiences in informed discourse by enabling them to 're-orientate their lives in wartime and understand the changing society around them'.[109] However, as our analysis of 'Fit to work' has indicated, the visual and textual language of the official film was far from radical, subordinating the citizen to professional expertise and endorsing conventional economic and social roles. *The Miner* issued a rebuff to traditional class relations, which may have also been palpable at factory showings where a majority were in skilled or semi-skilled manual jobs. Trade unionism, however, endorsed the other values that 'Fit to work' expounded: medical authority, heroic masculinity and the inevitable pathology of physical impairment. Of course, audiences spectated in a fragmented and not a monolithic way. Though mainly working-class, they differed in terms of occupation, gender, politics and national identity, and individual viewers negotiated their own readings of the film in the light of their personal beliefs and experiences.[110] None the less, the resulting 'myriad of meanings'[111] was constrained – though not determined – by the economic, social and political contexts in which production and consumption occurred.[112] It follows that the scope for advancing critical debate in an enlarged public sphere was limited. For whilst the documentary movement brought new issues to a wider public, their conservative representation discouraged the discussion of radical solutions. As social corporatism gained political credibility during the Second World War, so films like 'Fit to work' sought to sell its virtues to the masses, leaving unquestioned the underlying power relations between citizens and professionals, the economy and the state. In Habermas's terms, documentary audiences formed a 'culture-consuming' rather than a 'culture-debating' public.[113]

Notes

[1] Baxendale, J. and Pawling, C. (1996), *Narrating the Thirties: A Decade in the Making: 1930 to the Present* (Basingstoke, Macmillan), pp. 22–3, 26; Rotha, P. (1973), *Documentary Diary* (New York, Hill and Wang), pp. 20–1, 25.

[2] Hansen, M. (1993), 'Early cinema, late cinema: permutations of the public sphere', *Screen*, 34, 202.

[3] The Arts Enquiry (1947), *The Factual Film* (London, Oxford University Press), pp. 79–80; Thorpe, F. and Pronay, N. (1980), *British Official Films in the Second World War* (Oxford, Clio Press), pp. 256–63.

[4] Nichols, B. (1991), *Representing Reality: Issues and Concepts in Documentary* (Bloomington, Indiana University Press), pp. x, xiv. See also Corner, J. (1996), *The Art of the Record: A Critical Introduction to Documentary* (Manchester, Manchester University Press), pp. 1–3; Kilborn, R. and Izod, J. (1997), *An Introduction to Television Documentary: Confronting Reality* (Manchester, Manchester University Press), ch. 3; Pearson, D. (1982), 'Speaking for the common man: multi-voice commentary in *World of Plenty* and *Land of Promise*', in Marris, P. (ed.), *Paul Rotha*, BFI Dossier no. 16 (London, British Film Institute), pp. 71–2.

[5] Low, R. (1979), *Documentary and Educational Films of the 1930s* (London, George Allen and Unwin), p. 173.

[6] Rotha, *Documentary Diary*, pp. 16–17.

[7] Winston, B. (1995), *Claiming the Real: The Documentary Film Revisited* (London, British Film Institute), p. 11.

[8] Bruzzi, S. (2000), *New Documentary: A Critical Introduction* (London, Routledge), pp. 4, 6.

[9] Rotha, P. (1952), *Documentary Film* (London, Faber and Faber, first published 1935, 3rd edn), p. 88.

[10] Berry, D. (1994), *Wales and Cinema: The First Hundred Years* (Cardiff, University of Wales Press), pp. 137–8.

[11] Pronay, N. (1983), ' "The land of promise": the projection of peace aims in Britain', in Short, K. R. M. (ed.), *Film and Radio Propaganda in World War II* (London, Croom Helm), p. 68.

[12] Ibid., pp. 54–5. See also Thorpe and Pronay, *British Official Films*, p. 38.

[13] Forman, H. (1982), 'The non-theatrical distribution of films by the Ministry of Information', in Pronay, N. and Spring, D. W. (eds), *Propaganda, Politics and Film, 1918–1945* (London, Macmillan), p. 221. See also Thorpe and Pronay, *British Official Films*, p. 38.

[14] Parker, R. A. C. (1989), *Struggle for Survival: The History of the Second World War* (Oxford, Oxford University Press), p. 44.

[15] Chapman, J. (1998), *The British at War: Cinema, State and Propaganda, 1939–1945* (London, I. B. Tauris), pp. 20–1; Dickinson, M. and Street, S. (1985), *Cinema and State: The Film Industry and the State, 1927–1984* (London, British Film Institute), pp. 113–14; Thorpe and Pronay, *British Official Films*, p. 35.

[16] Forman, 'Non-theatrical distribution', pp. 232–3.

[17] Trevor Jones, A., Nixon, J. A. and Picken, R. M. F. (1945), *Hospital Survey: The Hospital Services of South Wales and Monmouthshire*, Welsh Board of Health (London, HMSO), p. 38. See also Titmuss, R. M. (1950), *Problems of Social Policy* (London, HMSO and Longmans, Green and Co.), p. 476.

[18] Newman, G. (1926), *An Outline of the Practice of Preventive Medicine: A Memorandum Addressed to the Minister of Health* (London, HMSO), p. 6.

[19] For a comprehensive discussion of these trends, and their implications for orthopaedics, see Cooter, R. (1993), *Surgery and Society in Peace and War: Orthopaedics and the Organization of Modern Medicine, 1880–1948* (Basingstoke, Macmillan), chs 4, 5, 8 and 9.

[20] Ibid., pp. 105, 141–2.

[21] Honigsbaum, F. (1979), *The Division in British Medicine: A History of the Separation of General Practice from Hospital Care, 1911–1968* (London, Kogan Page), p. 240.

[22] Titmuss, *Problems of Social Policy*, pp. 476–7.

[23] Jones, K. (1991), *The Making of Social Policy in Britain, 1830–1990* (London, Athlone), p. 120.

[24] Titmuss, *Problems of Social Policy*, pp. 477–8.

[25] Ibid., pp. 478–9.

[26] Jones, G. (1998), *The Aneurin Bevan Inheritance: The Story of the Nevill Hall and District NHS Trust* (Abertillery, Old Bakehouse Publications), p. 4.

[27] Richards, H. P. (1969), *A Short History of Caerphilly* (Caerphilly, Ellis Printers), p. 67.

[28] Caerphilly and District Miners' Hospital (1924), *Annual Report.*

[29] Ibid.

[30] Richards, *Short History of Caerphilly*, p. 67.

[31] Jenkins, P. (1992), *A History of Modern Wales, 1536–1990* (Harlow, Longman), p. 369.

[32] Caerphilly and District Miners' Hospital (1939), *Annual Report.*

[33] Caerphilly and District Miners' Hospital (1924), (1939), *Annual Reports*. The percentages for the second year exclude seventy patients admitted from the Glamorgan County Clinic.

[34] Jones, Nixon, and Picken, *Hospital Survey*, p. 57.

[35] Ibid.

[36] Newman, J. (1995), *Glamorgan* (Harmondsworth, Penguin Books), pp. 625–6; Ll. James, B. (1998), 'The making of a scholar ironmaster', in Ll. James, B. (ed.), *G. T. Clark: Scholar Ironmaster in the Victorian Age* (Cardiff, University of Wales Press), pp. 17–18; Croll, A. (1998), 'G. T. Clark, slums and sanitary reform', in James, *G. T. Clark*, pp. 24–42.

[37] *The Miner* (August 1946), 2.

[38] Hinton, J. (1983), *Labour and Socialism: A History of the British Labour Movement, 1867–1974* (Brighton, Wheatsheaf Books), pp. 110–12. The Sankey Commission found in favour of nationalization, and minimum hours and wages, but all these proposals were rejected by the government.

[39] Francis, H. and Smith, D. (1980), *The Fed: A History of the South Wales Miners in the Twentieth Century* (London, Lawrence and Wishart), p. 432; Hogenkamp, B. (1985), 'Miners' cinemas in south Wales in the 1920s and 1930s', *Llafur*, 4, 66; Nash, G. D., Davies, T. A. and Thomas, B. (1995), *Workmen's Halls and Institutes: Oakdale Workmen's Institute* (Cardiff, National Museums and Galleries of Wales), p. 10.

[40] *The Miner* (October/November 1946), 3.

[41] *The Miner* (June/July 1945), 18–19.

[42] *The Miner* (August 1946), 2–3.

[43] Ibid., 4.

[44] *The Miner* (June/July 1945), 20–1.

[45] *The Miner* (August 1945), 4–5.

[46] Jones, Nixon, and Picken, *Hospital Survey*, p. 38.

[47] Corner, *The Art of the Record*, pp. 65–6; Kilborn and Izod, *Introduction to Television Documentary*, pp. 5–6; Nichols, *Representing Reality*, p. 38.

[48] See also Winston, *Claiming the Real*, pp. 104–5.

[49] Kilborn and Izod, *Introduction to Television Documentary*, pp. 5–6; Nichols, *Representing Reality*, p. 38.

[50] Anderson, B. (1991), *Imagined Communities: Reflections on the Origins and Spread of Nationalism* (London, Verso, first published 1983; revised edn), p. 6.

[51] Fevre, R. and Thompson, A. (1999), 'Social theory and Welsh identities', in Fevre, R. and Thompson, A., *Nation, Identity and Social Theory: Perspectives from Wales* (Cardiff, University of Wales Press), pp. 5, 12.

[52] Stead, P. (1988), 'The people as stars: feature films as national expression', in Taylor, P. M. (ed.), *Britain and the Cinema in the Second World War* (Basingstoke, Macmillan), p. 65.

[53] Jackson, K. (1995), 'Images of the Industrial Revolution, 1660–1886: Humphrey Jennings and *Pandaemonium*', unpublished paper delivered to a conference of the Society for the Social History of Medicine entitled 'Industrialization and public health: redrawing the picture', held at the Science Museum, 6–7.

[54] Berry, *Wales and Cinema*, pp. 137–40, 150, 160–2, 187–8, 191, 457–8.

[55] Lewis, R. (1996), 'The Welsh radical tradition and the ideal of a democratic popular culture', in Biagini, E. F. (ed.), *Citizenship and Community: Liberals, Radicals and Collective Identities in the British Isles, 1865–1931* (Cambridge,

Cambridge University Press), pp. 327–9, 332, 335, 339–40. See also Adamson, D. (1999), 'The intellectual and national movement in Wales', in Fevre and Thompson, *Nation, Identity and Social Theory*, pp. 48–67.

[56] Gruffudd, P. (1995), '"A crusade against consumption": environment, health and social reform in Wales, 1900–1939', *Journal of Historical Geography*, 21, 49–50.

[57] *The Miner* (August 1946), 14. See also *The Miner* (October 1946). Men sawing wood were used to demonstrate artificial limbs in a short 1918 film of the opening ceremony of the Prince of Wales Orthopaedic Hospital in Cardiff. See Wales Film and Television Archive, video no. FOF1 611.

[58] *The Miner* (August 1946), 2. See also *Convalescent Home for the South Wales Mining Industry, Pontyclun* (publisher and exact date of publication unknown), Foreword.

[59] Cooter, *Surgery and Society*, pp. 187, 195, 218. See also Barsam, R. M. (1992), *Non-Fiction Film: A Critical History* (Bloomington and Indianapolis, Indiana University Press), p. 194; Colls, R. and Dodd, P. (1985), 'Representing the nation: British documentary film, 1930–1945', *Screen*, 26, 21; Titmuss, *Problems of Social Policy*, pp. 476, 480.

[60] Aitken, I. (1989), 'John Grierson, idealism and the inter-war period', *Historical Journal of Film, Radio and Television*, 9, 247–56; Baxendale and Pawling, *Narrating the Thirties*, pp. 25–9; Parker, J. (1998), *Citizenship, Work and Welfare: Searching for the Good Society* (Basingstoke, Macmillan), p. 125.

[61] Aiken, *John Grierson*, pp. 247–50, 254–6; Kilborn and Izod, *Introduction to Television Documentary*, pp. 30–2.

[62] Bynum, W. F. (1994), *Science and the Practice of Medicine in the Nineteenth Century* (Cambridge, Cambridge University Press), pp. 221–2.

[63] Bury, M. (1998), 'Postmodernity and health', in Scambler, G. and Higgs, P. (eds), *Modernity, Medicine and Health: Medical Sociology towards 2000* (London, Routledge), pp. 5–6. See also Fissell, M. E. (1991) 'The disappearance of the patient's narrative and the invention of hospital medicine', in French, R. and Wear, A. (eds), *British Medicine in an Age of Reform* (London, Routledge), pp. 92–109.

[64] Cooter, *Surgery and Society*, p. 187.

[65] Honigsbaum, *Division in British Medicine*, pp. 239–41.

[66] Featherstone, M. (1992), 'The heroic and everyday life', *Theory, Culture and Society*, 9, 162.

[67] *The Miner* (October 1944), 8–9.

[68] *The Miner* (August 1946), 6–13.

[69] Colls and Dodd, 'Representing the nation', 29.

[70] Giddens, A. (1991) *Modernity and Self-Identity: Self and Society in the Late Modern Age* (Cambridge, Polity Press), pp. 161–2.

[71] Rotha, *Documentary Film*, p. 97; Rotha, *Documentary Diary*, p. 28; Barsam, *Non-Fiction Film*, pp. 82, 90, 96, 99, 189.

[72] Colls and Dodd, 'Representing the nation', 22–3.

[73] Ibid., 23; Corner, J. *The Art of the Record*, p. 70.

[74] Colls and Dodd, 'Representing the nation', 32.

[75] *Convalescent Home for the South Wales Mining Industry*, Foreword. See also *The Miner* (August 1946), 2–3.

[76] *The Miner* (October 1946), 4–5.

[77] Ibid., 4, 16.

[78] For a discussion of this problem in the late nineteenth and early twentieth

centuries, see Jones, D. (1991), 'Counting the cost of coal: women's lives in the Rhondda, 1881–1911', in John, A. V. (ed.), *Our Mothers' Land: Chapters in Welsh Women's History, 1830–1939* (Cardiff, University of Wales Press), pp. 109–33.

[79] Braybon, G. and Summerfield, P. (1987), *Out of the Cage: Women's Experiences in Two World Wars* (London, Pandora), pp. 237–8.

[80] Harper, S. (1988), 'The representation of women in British feature films, 1939–45', in Taylor, P. M. (ed.), *Britain and the Cinema in the Second World War* (Basingstoke, Macmillan), pp. 170–1, 173–6.

[81] Colls and Dodd, 'Representing the nation', 24–5; Corner, *The Art of the Record*, pp. 61–3.

[82] Miles, P. and Smith, M. (1987), *Cinema, Literature and Society: Elite and Mass Culture in Interwar Britain* (London, Croom Helm), pp. 189–91.

[83] See also Barsam, *Non-Fiction Film*, p. 107.

[84] *The Miner* (August 1946), 14.

[85] Hughes, G. (1998), 'A suitable case for treatment? Constructions of disability', in Saraga, E. (ed.), *Embodying the Social: Constructions of Difference* (London, Routledge and the Open University), p. 79. See also Abberley, P. (1996), 'Work, utopia and impairment', in Barton, L. (ed.), *Disability and Society: Emerging Issues and Insights* (Harlow, Longman), pp. 74–5.

[86] *The Miner* (October 1946), 14–15.

[87] Hogenkamp, 'Miners' cinemas', 67.

[88] Humphries, S. and Gordon, P. (1992), *Out of Sight: The Experience of Disability, 1900–1950* (Plymouth, Northcote House), pp. 129–36.

[89] Ibid., pp. 134–5.

[90] Oliver, M. and Barnes, C. (1998), *Disabled People and Social Policy: From Exclusion to Inclusion* (Harlow, Longman), pp. 3–6, 49. See also Oliver, M. (1990), *The Politics of Disablement* (Basingstoke, Macmillan), pp. 9–11, 22–4, 78–94; Borsay, A. (1986), 'Personal trouble or public issue? Towards a model of policy for people with physical and mental disabilities', *Disability, Handicap and Society*, 1, 179–95.

[91] UPIAS (1976), *Fundamental Principles of Disability* (London, Union of the Physically Impaired against Segration), p. 4.

[92] This debate is effectively addressed in Barnes, C. and Mercer, G. (eds) (1996), *Exploring the Divide: Illness and Disability* (Leeds, Disability Press).

[93] Shearer, A. (1981), *Disability: Whose Handicap?* (Oxford, Blackwell), p. 7.

[94] Parker, *Citizenship, Work and Welfare*, pp. 146–7.

[95] See, for example, Borsay, A. (1986), *Disabled People in the Community: A Study of Housing, Health and Welfare Services* (London, Bedford Square Press); Buckle, J. R. (1971), *Work and Housing of Impaired Persons in Great Britain* (London, HMSO); Harris, A. I., Cox, E. and Smith, C. R. W. (1971), *Handicapped and Impaired in Great Britain* (London, HMSO); Sainsbury, S. (1970), *Registered as Disabled* (London, Bell).

[96] Nixon, S. (1997), 'Exhibiting masculinity', in Hall, S. (ed.), *Representation: Cultural Representations and Signifying Practices* (London, Sage and the Open University), p. 302.

[97] Baxendale and Pawling, *Narrating the Thirties*, p. 37.

[98] Chapman, *The British at War*, p. 86.

[99] Pronay, ' "The land of promise" ', p. 72.

[100] Barsam, *Non-Fiction Film*, p. 98.

[101] Thorpe and Pronay, *British Official Films*, pp. 37–8.

[102] The Arts Enquiry, *The Factual Film*, p. 79.

[103] Chapman, *The British at War*, pp. 45–6, 87, 107–8.

[104] Barsam, *Non-Fiction Film*, p. 189.

[105] Fredlund, L. and Marris, P. (1982), 'Interview: Rotha on Rotha', in Marris, (ed.), *Paul Rotha*, p. 25.

[106] Winston, *Claiming the Real*, p. 35; Barsam, *Non-Fiction Film*, p. 189.

[107] Fredlund and Marris, 'Interview', p. 25.

[108] The Arts Enquiry, *The Factual Film*, p. 83; Forman, 'Non-theatrical distribution', pp. 227, 231–2.

[109] Forman, 'Non-theatrical distribution', 223–4.

[110] Chapman, *The British at War*, pp. 252–4; Rodowick, D. N. (1994), *The Crisis of Political Modernism: Criticism and Ideology in Contemporary Film Theory* (Berkeley, University of California Press), pp. xxiv–xxv.

[111] Allen, R.C. (1990), 'From exhibition to reception: reflections on the audience in film history', *Screen*, 31, 353.

[112] Allen, R. C. and Gomery, D. (1985), *Film History: Theory and Practice* (New York, McGraw-Hill), p. 170.

[113] Habermas, J. (1989), *The Structural Transformation of the Public Sphere* (Cambridge, Polity Press), pp. 159–75.

8

Private Lives and Public Bodies: Childbirth in Post-war Swansea

❧

SUSAN J. PITT

Introduction

This chapter is based on evidence gained during an oral history project carried out with doctors and midwives who were practising in the Swansea area between 1945 and 1974, as well as evidence from medical and midwifery textbooks published in the same period. It is argued that no simple relationship can be made between the public/private dichotomy and gender. Within the context of childbirth in the post-war period, there was a masculinization of both public and private spheres. In the public sphere, changing conceptions of district and community led to an undermining of the autonomous role of the district midwife as the hospital consultant became the central figure. In the private sphere, the woman-to-woman relationships between the extended family and female neighbours were eroded as the nuclear family became the basic unit of society. This led to the entry of the father into the delivery room, despite him being seen as 'a stranger in with the delivery' by many of the older midwives. Furthermore, developments in techniques of visualization during pregnancy and monitoring during labour increasingly meant that the birthing woman's body itself was no longer private. It is concluded that this process of masculinization was the cause of the discomfort which led many women to complain about their experience of birth in the 1970s and 1980s.

Gender and the Public/Private Dichotomy

Our language and our traditions almost inevitably lead us to make assumptions about gender as soon as we begin to discuss the public and the private because there is a structured association between the private sphere and the feminine and between the public sphere and the masculine. Although those associations are in no way necessary or inevitable, they operate at such a deep level in our consciousness that we have to work hard to question them. Historians of gender have already carried out some of this questioning work, most notably Leonore Davidoff and Catherine Hall, who point out the complexity of the relationship between gender and the public/private dichotomy in their work on the nineteenth-century family.[1] It is this questioning work which I aim to continue here. When we look in detail at an area such as childbirth, what we find is an extremely complex set of ideas about the public and the private which are certainly gendered, but not in any simple way.

Most of the modern history of childbirth revolves around the big issue of the 'male take-over' – of how and why childbirth was transformed from an entirely female preserve in the seventeenth century into a highly medicalized, technologized and masculinized experience at the end of the twentieth century. It would be easy to see this process of masculinization as simply linked to the public/ private dichotomy: traditional childbirth was a private female event, while modern childbirth has been made all too public for the comfort of many birthing women. Yet it is clear if we look at the work of Adrian Wilson that birth has always been a public event. In fact, the main role of the female 'gossips' who attended birth in the seventeenth century was to 'witness' the birth – to act on behalf of society to ensure that this really was the child of this woman, that this child was dead at birth and not smothered by its mother, and so on.[2] It is also clear that late twentieth-century childbirth could be seen in some ways as more private than traditional child-birth – it is now firmly based within the nuclear family rather than the extended community of traditional birth. Yet it remains true that many women, particularly in the 1970s and 1980s, reacted very strongly against their experience of birth – they felt violated, they felt that what should have been a private event under their own control was in fact taken out of their hands and made into a public event which they could not control. If we are to understand why this was the case, we need to look beyond the conventional 'male take-over' story which focuses entirely on the sex of the practitioners – female midwives displaced by male doctors – and look instead at gender as a complex cultural construction. This means that we must consider relationships and processes rather than individuals.

There are two key issues here. Firstly, we need to consider that what is understood by the terms public and private might change historically. It is clear, for example, that there was a profound change in understandings of the 'public' during and after the Second World War. There is an ongoing debate amongst historians about the extent to which the post-war welfare state was built upon a 'consensus' around the idea of taking collective responsibility for the welfare of every member of society.[3] This very debate highlights the extent to which notions of public and private responsibility were being renegotiated at this time. Here I will be arguing that part of that process of renegotiation entailed a rethinking of understandings of family and community which significantly changed the relationships of power between women and their birth attendants, and between women and other members of the family/ community.

Secondly, we need to look at the micropolitics of power which governed these gendered interactions between birthing women and their attendants. Under the National Health Service, the collective responsibility for bringing healthy babies into the world was mediated by the professions of medicine and midwifery. Elsewhere I have argued that during the post-war period the discourse of midwifery was gradually superseded by the discourse of medicine. The effect of this was to displace the discourse of midwifery which had held sway in normal births and to replace it with a medically dominated discourse which assumed an ever-present risk of abnormality even if none was so far apparent. By the mid-1970s, both midwives and doctors were practising in ways which were structured by the discourse of medicine.[4] Embedded in this medical discourse, there was an imperative to 'know' the birthing woman in a particular way – in an objective, distancing way which made the events of pregnancy and birth transparent, public, there for all to see. So if we are to understand women's feelings of discomfort with their experiences of birth, we need to look in detail at the practices of midwives and doctors in this period.

This chapter falls into two parts. I will start with a discussion of changing understandings of community and family within the context of childbirth practices in the post-war period. This is based on an oral history project carried out in 1992 and 1993. In-depth interviews were held with nineteen doctors and midwives who had provided maternity care in Swansea between 1945 and 1974. The sample was gathered by the snowball technique, and the interviews were taped and transcribed.[5] The second part of the chapter will be about the changing management of childbirth in the same period. This evidence comes from analysis of medical and midwifery textbooks published at the time. Although it does not relate specifically to Wales, the textbooks were very widely used and hence there is a very good chance that my sample of professionals had been influenced by them.[6]

Constructing the Public and the Private: Community and Family

So to begin with the discussion of community and family. In the period immediately after the Second World War, all midwives working from their own homes became known as 'district midwives'. By the 1970s they had become 'community midwives'. I think this signified a profound change in the way in which communities were understood – the way in which the public was understood. When the National Health Service was introduced, hospital births fell under the organizational umbrella of the Regional Hospital Boards, but the responsibility for home-based midwifery and for maternal and child welfare work remained with the local authorities. With the reorganization of 1974 the service was unified and brought under the control of the new Regional Health Boards. The effect of this was that the midwife ceased to be seen as a relatively autonomous figure in a local district and instead became a community outreach worker in what was essentially a hospital-based service. This made an important difference to the way she related to the birthing woman.

It was the older district midwives who demonstrated a particularly strong sense of being part of the local 'district' in both a geographical and a social sense. As Nurse Lillian Morgan put it: 'And I bought a house on Townhill Road by the college. Semi-detached. I was there, I was up on the hill for thirty one years doing my midwifery.[7] Women would simply come round to the house when they knew they were pregnant, or would seek antenatal care in an even more informal way, as Nurse Janey Jones described: 'But some, of course, some of my patients, I'd meet them in Woolworth's and they'd say "Nurse, be wanting you soon", you know [laughs]. I'd try and chase them up then, you know.'[8] These midwives lived within a district and were already well known by those who became pregnant.

Nurse Janey Jones later went to work in Fairwood Hospital and she missed the familiarity with local people as a result:

> My name went round as Nurse Janey. I was never called Nurse Jones. When I went to Fairwood the matron was rather annoyed about that . . . And the kiddies used to call out, shout out 'Nurse Janey' to me, you know on the street. You know, most of them were my babies. No, it was a very happy time, I enjoyed all that district work, really happy. I was much happier on district really, than in hospital, because you were, it was impersible, imperson somehow, you know.[9]

There was, then, a strong sense of personal involvement in the lives of generations of people living in her district which she felt was less easily expressed in the hospital environment.

Another of my interviewees, Sister Gerty Morgan, showed a similarly strong sense of involvement with the local community, despite the fact that she worked as a hospital midwife throughout her career. She had read in the paper of the death of a local man:

> And they gave names of the family left, his wife, his daughter. I delivered his wife of the daughter. And then the daughter's name was there, and I delivered her. And I thought 'Well goodness me. All those people, I delivered those.' The grandmother you see, the grandmother, the mother and the daughter.

The wedding of a local woman was reported in the paper:

> And now she was a singer up in London somewhere. She went to college and that and she qualified and she's a marvellous singer. And there were huge pictures in the Evening Post, and I looked and I thought 'Well well well, to think I delivered you'. And she lived in the little house

in Birch Grove, a little cottage – village up from Llansamlet, and just an ordinary mother and father, you know? And – she's an only child. I remember the, I remember the *day* she was delivered, there was such a fuss, she was the only one. And then these beautiful, these beautiful pictures, from the cathedral, oh dear.[10]

This sense of belonging to a social network was particularly marked in her as a Welsh-speaker, but it is significant that the events she picked out were those of birth, marriage and death. This highlights the sense of the midwife as the guardian of just one of the rites of passage that were important in a local district. So despite the fact that she worked in hospital, she still had that involvement with 'the district' – although her district would have been more extensive than that of a district midwife.

The real contrast comes between these older midwives and a much younger midwife – Nurse Lillian Smith – who was still working as a community midwife at the time of the interview. She had a strong sense of community, but it was expressed rather differently. She explained how, because she had worked in the area for so long, her knowledge of local people could be useful to other health-care practitioners, such as the health visitors, with whom she now shared an office.[11] This highlights the sense of her being part of the system of surveillance in the local community, while the older midwives were more like traditional wise women. There was still a feeling of close involvement with the community, as evidenced by a local charity raising money to provide her with a sonic aid.[12] This was, however, a very particular kind of functional gift-giving which can be contrasted to the way in which Nurse Lillian Morgan was given a set of fish knives and forks by a woman she had delivered who had heard that she herself was getting married.[13] The fact that the cutlery was carefully kept and never used indicates the non-functional nature of the gift – it served to incorporate the midwife into a network of social relations and to mark an important rite of passage for her, rather than being something she would use in her work.

Several of the general practitioners revealed a similar sense of district to that of the older midwives. As Dr A. Law explained:

I must say that our practice population are very loyal to us, having had, having had perhaps five generations in the one practice there is a kind of loyalty. And we don't discourage people from staying with the practice, even though they move out to the peripheral estates.

Later on he added:

> And with the kind of practice that I have tried to convey to you it was, we were looking after the children and the grandchildren of people who had been confined in the practice, you see. And in fact, although we do very little, we do virtually no home obstetrics now, of course, but from an antenatal point of view, I've seen the children and sometimes even the grandchildren of people I looked after antenatally – in the early days. So there's this kind of, kind of trust and support that, that you get from a family practice of this kind.[14]

Dr Baker also saw involvement in childbirth as a way of cementing his position within social networks:

> Looking after the babies was – a real start of family doctoring wasn't it? You know, you got to know the patients and – there's a bond formed between you and a definite rapport with a pregnant woman, and especially when she's had the baby, and hopefully everything went okay, and thank goodness nearly always it did, and you had a rapport, and it's a good way of doing general practice.[15]

This shows a very similar sense of involvement over generations to that demonstrated by Sister Gerty Morgan, but general practitioners no longer took any significant part in birth itself from the 1970s onwards – virtually all births then took place in hospital. And the hospital consultants I interviewed showed very little sense of being involved in the local community – they had their own social networks but these were very separate from their interaction with patients within the hospital.

So what is happening over time is that the sense of GPs and midwives being part of a particular district is displaced by a new sense of community which is centred on the hospital and with the community midwives and GPs acting as a kind of surveillance system on behalf of the consultant. This sets up a much more distant relationship between the birthing woman and her attendants in birth. 'The public' is no longer the local district which is the woman's home, but is now centred on the hospital. The woman is no longer attended by a midwife and GP who are part of her own social network, but by public figures who are at one step removed from her.

Another important change which was associated with this was that the birthing woman came to be seen as centred in the nuclear family. The result was that the father took over the role of lay witness to the birth which had been performed by the gossips in the seventeenth century and by female relatives or neighbours more recently. This can be seen as part of a wider social process in which the extended family was becoming more separate and the nuclear family was becoming the basic unit of society. Michael Young and Peter Willmott have referred to this new unit as the 'symmetrical family' which arose as the informal 'woman's trade union' broke down.[16] As 'district' was reconfigured as 'community', then, childbirth became less of a female preserve and more the concern of a nuclear family. And the female relative or neighbour who had previously attended the birth was now displaced by the father of the child.

It was not until the mid-1960s that it became at all usual for the father of the child to be present in the delivery room. This meant that for many of the professionals I interviewed the presence of the father was a controversial issue. Those who continued to practise in the 1970s and 1980s became more accepting of his presence, and it is clear that this results from a new way of thinking about family. As Sister Hughes put it: 'And I mean, I suppose that it is a family affair, so why not? It's theirs as well as the mother's.'[17] It was this notion of the nuclear family rather than the extended family or the wider social group that Nurse Janey Jones was promoting when she said that she thought it was a good thing to have fathers present:

> Get them involved with it, with the mother and the baby I always used to say. And when I was in Fairwood I used to encourage them to, to come there into the labour ward, we used to let them. And another thing was, when the mother was going out and that, the grandmother would always want to carry the baby, but I would always give it to the husband, for him to carry. Get him involved with the baby straight away I reckoned.[18]

Here we can really see how the female member of the extended family is being displaced by the father.

Many of the older midwives, however, continued to see the father as a problematic presence during childbirth. He was accused of interfering in the relationship between woman and midwife and of undermining the midwife's authority. Those midwives who had had grudgingly to accept the presence of the father often spoke of him in very derogatory ways. I was told innumerable stories which revealed the incompetence of the father, and of course the mythology of the father fainting at the sight of blood remains with us today. I think that much of this negative attitude towards the father derived from a sense that he was in some way out of place in the delivery room. Many of the older midwives mentioned quite specifically that they felt that the privacy of the birth was being invaded by the father. Sister Gerty Morgan tried to ensure that fathers were not allowed into the delivery rooms in Morriston Hospital at all until she retired in 1968. As she explained: 'I always thought it was something, perhaps I was old fashioned, I thought it was more private for the mother.'[19] Sister Howell, despite having come to accept their presence, described fathers as 'a stranger in with the delivery', and said that her personal preference was for the father to come in after the delivery: 'I think that is rather nice myself, in my opinion. You know, when the patient has been sponged down and put comfortable and the baby's been cleaned up a bit.'[20]

Even some midwives who were generally positive about fathers in the delivery room expressed clear views about what they should and should not be allowed to see. As Sister Hughes put it: 'Occasionally you would have somebody who would decide to go down and have a look see what was going on at the bottom end, and he was – usually sent back to the top end where he – should be.'[21] So even when the father was admitted to the room, the midwife was concerned that the father should not observe the actual birth. This can be contrasted with the role which female relatives had previously been expected to play. There was no real sense of them being in the wrong place, especially with home deliveries. They were not barred from the 'bottom end', and Dr A. Law even suggested that the mother of the labouring woman could hold one knee while he held the other as the midwife conducted the second stage.[22] It was also assumed that they would play a useful role. Nurse Thomas relied on the mother to bring water for her and Dr W. O. Williams declared: 'Oh I don't mind if they can have a female relative if they help, if they do something to help the midwife.' Dr W. O. Williams followed this comment up with a story about a delivery which he had had to deal with on his own before the midwife managed to reach the house and in which the grandmother had lain curled up – apparently asleep – in the same bed as the labouring woman throughout the proceedings. This meant that he was deprived of all female assistance, with the result that he got in a terrible mess and dropped the placenta on the floor.[23] This is in complete contrast to fathers who were assumed to be incapable of helping at all.

So what I have suggested is that the change from 'district' to 'community' in the post-war period changed understandings of the public. The district had been a local social network in which both birthing woman and medical and midwifery practitioners were embedded. The community was much more distant – it was centred on the hospital and the practitioners were anonymous figures from a separate social network to that of the birthing woman. Furthermore, that community was composed of separate nuclear families, headed by fathers, rather than the extended network of female relatives and neighbours which had dominated within the district. The presence of the father in the delivery room was a natural outcome of this shift, but was seen by many of the older practitioners as an invasion of the privacy of the birth. The fact that the father is now seen as the most appropriate witness to the birth shows how far our understandings of privacy have shifted. It is clear that both of these shifts entailed a masculinization of birth – the increasing dominance of the hospital consultant and the displacement of female relatives by the father. This process of masculinization becomes even more apparent if we turn to look at the actual management of birth.

Constructing the Public and the Private: Women's Bodies Made Public

I will start with a discussion of monitoring, which is one area which has been very contentious. In particular, controversy has focused on the use of electronic monitors to record the foetal heart rate and to measure the strength of uterine contractions because this restricts the movements of the labouring woman and makes her passive. These were both techniques which were introduced in the 1970s, but it is clear from the textbooks that monitoring was being carried out by midwives for many years before this without women complaining about it.

In midwifery textbooks of the late 1940s and early 1950s, midwives were told of the importance of 'Observation of the woman in labour'.[24] Obstetrics textbooks from the same period made no mention of any kind of monitoring during labour, so monitoring was clearly not a concern for doctors at this time. It is worth looking in some detail at how midwives carried out this process. The following extract is taken from a midwifery textbook published in 1953:

> A record of the progress of labour should be faithfully kept, both in hospital and in the home. The frequency, duration, and strength of contractions should be recorded at regular intervals of not more than 2 hours, and more frequently, particularly towards the end of the first stage, if there is any cause for anxiety. At the same time, the descent of the presenting part should be estimated, and the rate and regularity of the foetal heart sounds and the mother's pulse rate should be recorded. The temperature should be taken 4-hourly and the blood-pressure 8-hourly, and if the labour is slow the urine should be tested for acetone. The bladder must be kept empty, and a record kept of the amount of urine passed. If labour passes into a second or even a third day, the advisability of repeating the enema daily must be considered. The time at which the membranes rupture should be recorded, and the liquor observed to see whether it contains meconium or not.
>
> Rectal or vaginal examinations may be necessary (with all the necessary precautions taken against infection) to assess the progress of labour, *i.e.* the dilatation of the os uteri and the descent of the presenting part, but abdominal examination should first be made, and internal examinations only if necessary to confirm the abdominal findings.
>
> It is highly important to note the effect of the second-stage contractions upon both mother and foetus. The maternal pulse rate and foetal heart sounds must be checked every quarter of an hour. An increase in the mother's pulse rate with or without a rise of temperature will be one of the first indications of some distress on the part of the mother. The increase or decrease of the foetal heart sounds is a sign of foetal distress. Later, meconium may be passed.[25]

This reveals that detailed monitoring of labour was being carried out by the midwife, but there are some important points to note. Firstly, it is the '*woman* in labour' who is being observed. Most of the indicators are to be seen in the woman herself: it is her pulse, her blood pressure, her level of distress which reassure the midwife that everything is progressing normally. Uterine contractions were assessed simply by the midwife laying her hand on the labouring woman's abdomen, and the reluctance to carry out the more invasive vaginal or rectal examinations is clear. Although the midwife is clearly concerned about the well-being of the foetus, foetal distress is seen as a corollary of maternal distress. The foetal heart sounds were heard through a foetal stethoscope, which entailed a degree of intimacy between midwife and labouring woman as compared to the more distancing effect of the later electronic monitoring.[26] This monitoring, then, focused primarily on the birthing woman, seeing her interests as coinciding with those of the baby. The other important point is that the midwife was simply observing the course of normal labour and looking out for abnormality should it arise. She was noting when the membranes ruptured rather than breaking them artificially, and the labour was seen as having its own rhythm and rate of progress. It was assumed that the labour would simply take its course and the midwife only had to worry if a definite abnormality occurred.

This can be contrasted with the form of monitoring which appears in both midwifery and obstetrics texts from the late 1960s. New time limits were set for labour. In the 1972 edition of the midwifery textbook quoted above, the section on monitoring in labour made no mention of 'slow' labours, and the possibility of a labour continuing into a second or third day was not even considered.[27] The progress of labour was now to be recorded in graph form, as a 'partogram', so that it could at any stage be compared with the 'normal' trajectory for labour. It was now assumed that the partogram allowed the practitioner to read off the degree of cervical dilatation which should have occurred after a given number of hours of labour, the time at which the second stage should begin, as well as the time by which delivery should be complete. What is interesting about this is that the older process of monitoring assumed a kind of integrity of the woman's body – it was carrying on with labour in its own way and only under certain clearly defined circumstances would the labour be considered 'abnormal'. With the new approach there was an established conception of what labour should be like – there was a public standard against which a woman's labour could be judged.

By the 1970s the electronic monitoring of uterine contractions and the foetal heart rate had been introduced. This allowed the production of a continuous trace which revealed any increase or decrease in the foetal heart rate and showed how any such changes related to the timing of contractions. It is noteworthy that the chapter on this subject in the 1972 edition of *Obstetrics by Ten Teachers* is entitled 'The Fetus at Risk'.[28] For obstetricians, the development of electronic monitoring of both the foetal heart and the mother's uterine contractions aimed solely to ensure the well-being of the foetus. This means that rather than monitoring being carried out to ensure the well-being of the woman (and therefore her child), in the later obstetrics texts monitoring is about keeping a public eye on the performance of the woman in labour so that the interests of her unborn child could be protected. This effectively undermines any sense that the baby is still part of its mother's body – her body is no longer allowed to be private. It is not monitoring as such which leads to discomfort, it is monitoring carried out in a particular way and with a particular purpose which invades the woman's sense of privacy.

A similar invasion occurs with the use of technologies of visualization, such as X-ray and ultrasound. In the immediate post-war period, X-ray was the only technique available. This was used only where a particular abnormality was suspected. In 1958 a link was established between antenatal radiography and childhood cancer deaths. This coincided with the time at which ultrasound was being developed, so that as X-rays were abandoned a new technique was there to take its place. Ultrasound was first used clinically in 1960 and was being recommended for routine use by 1980.[29]

There has been a strong feminist critique of the use of ultra-sound. Ann Oakley, for example, has argued that the technique allowed obstetricians to see through what they saw as the 'veritable iron curtain' of the mother's abdomen so that they no longer had to rely on what the mother thought or felt in order to obtain information on the foetus. This resulted in the foetus becoming the central focus of obstetric interest while the mother became irrelevant; a mere 'walking womb'.[30] These ideas have been elaborated by Rosalind Pollack Petchesky who has commented on the power of ultrasound images in a visually oriented culture such as our own. She has argued that while the photographic image gives the impression of being objective, it also has mythical qualities:

> The autonomous, free-floating foetus merely extends to gestation the Hobbesian view of born human beings as disconnected, solitary individuals. It is this abstract individualism, effacing the pregnant woman and the foetus' dependence on her, that gives the foetal image its symbolic transparency.[31]

She goes on to argue that technologies of visualization have the effect of disrupting definitions of what is inside of and outside of a woman's body: 'treating a foetus *as if it were* outside a woman's body, because it can be viewed, is a political act.'[32] The making public of the foetus undermines the pregnant woman's control over what is happening in that most private of places – her own body.

It is clear that the development of ultrasound as a means of assessing foetal development and well-being changed the bodily interactions between pregnant women and their attendants in important ways. Early in this period, the size of the uterus was assessed by its position in relation to parts of the woman's body and was measured as being so many fingers' breadth away from the umbilicus or symphysis pubis. The abdominal girth could also be measured with a tape measure or with callipers.[33] The foetal heart was heard through a foetal stethoscope. Such techniques were to some extent eclipsed by the development of ultrasound in the 1960s and 1970s, although midwives still placed emphasis on the value of the older techniques. Ultrasound could be used to measure the increasing size of the foetal skull and the foetal heart could be 'heard' without use of the foetal stethoscope by the use of the Doppler effect.[34]

This change in the technologies used to assess foetal development changed the bodily interactions between the woman and her attendants. The earlier techniques saw foetal development as an intrinsic part of the woman's body, and it was her body which showed the signs which could be monitored. The midwife's body was used in intimate ways as her hands were laid on the woman's abdomen and her ear was held close to the foetal stethoscope. 'Listening' to the foetal heart by the later technique means that the midwife remains standing at the side of the pregnant woman and simply holds the transducer against her abdomen – a much more distant interaction. The later techniques rendered the mother's body irrelevant; it simply had to be penetrated in order to observe the foetus. It was the foetus which had to be made public – it was no longer to be confined within the private space of the woman's body – that space was no longer private.

To take the argument still further, according to Ludmilla Jordanova, there are particularly sexual connotations to the medical desire for visualization.[35] This is confirmed by the fact that in the nineteenth century men-midwives were allowed to touch women patients but not see them, suggesting that vision was even more violating than touch.[36] This means that the use of ultrasound can be seen as symbolically sexually penetrative. Yet the textbooks reveal that the desire to penetrate the woman's body visually was not an entirely new phenomenon. Ultrasound in many ways simply took the place of X-rays in antenatal diagnosis. Importantly, however, X-ray was seen as appropriate only when abnormality of various kinds was suspected. This was to change as new ways of thinking about pregnancy and labour were developed in the 1970s – all pregnancies now required visual surveillance because they were all now deemed to be potentially abnormal. It was ultrasound which took on this role of routine surveillance of all pregnancies.[37] The importance of ultrasound, then, was not just that it entailed a sexual violation of the woman's body – X-rays did so too – but that it constituted bodies which were *always* open to that violation in order to keep them on the normal trajectory rather than only in response to abnormality.

So what we are seeing in both the monitoring of labour and in the techniques of visualization in pregnancy is a shift in focus away from the birthing woman and towards the unborn child. Instead of it being assumed that there is an integrity of the woman/baby unit, with the interests of the baby being utterly entwined with those of its mother, increasingly the woman's body is seen almost as an obstacle which gets in the way of the obstetrician's desire to protect the interests of the baby. The woman's body is measured in a distancing 'objective' way and compared to a public standard, and the contents of her womb are no longer privately enclosed in that body – they are made public so that collective responsibility can be taken for them.

Conclusion

So to conclude, then: what I have been arguing is that there is no simple relationship between the public/private dichotomy and gender. In the context of childbirth in post-war Swansea, I have identified a process of masculinization of both public and private spheres. As 'district' was reconfigured into 'community', the district midwife lost her autonomy as the hospital consultant became the central figure – a masculinization of the public sphere. As female relatives and neighbours were displaced by the father in the delivery room, that private space was also masculinized. And as the medical imperatives for monitoring and visualization became routine even in normal pregnancies, that most private of places – the woman's own body – was made public in the most masculine of ways. I believe that it was this process of masculinization which left women feeling such discomfort at their experience of birth. It is interesting to consider how childbirth practitioners have responded to women's complaints about their treatment during pregnancy and labour in the period since the early 1980s. One response has been the attempt to recreate a homely private space for birth by putting curtains and carpets, wallpaper and easy chairs into hospital delivery rooms. Yet this increased 'privacy' does little to ease women's discomfort when the practices of birth attendants (both doctors and midwives) remain governed by the masculinist discourse of medicine. Whilst most women choose to give birth in hospital and willingly submit to the processes of monitoring, many of them are left with feelings of failure and of violation afterwards. If we are to make a real difference to this, we need to look beyond the fixed dichotomies of female midwife versus male doctor, public versus private, and begin a process of feminization.

Notes

[1] Davidoff, L. and Hall, C. (1987), *Family Fortunes: Men and Women of the English Middle Class 1780–1850* (London, Hutchinson).

[2] Wilson, A. (1995), *The Making of the Man-Midwife: Childbirth in England, 1660–1770* (Cambridge, MA, Harvard University Press), p. 25.

[3] For a summary of the debate see Smith, M. (1993), 'The changing nature of the British state, 1929–59: the historiography of consensus', in Brivati, B. and Jones, H. (eds), *What Difference did the War Make?* (London, Leicester University Press), pp. 37–47.

[4] Pitt, S. (1996), 'Midwifery and medicine: discourses in childbirth, c. 1945–1974' (unpublished Ph.D. thesis, University of Wales, Lampeter).

[5] Ibid., 6–7.

[6] Ibid., 11.

[7] Interview with Nurse Lillian Morgan carried out by S. Pitt on 3 June 1992.

[8] Interview with Nurse Janey Jones carried out by S. Pitt on 2 October 1992.

[9] Interview with Nurse Janey Jones.

[10] Interview with Sister Gerty Morgan carried out by S. Pitt on 13 October 1992.

[11] Interview with Nurse Lillian Smith carried out by S. Pitt on 23 October 1992.

[12] Interview with Nurse Lillian Smith.

[13] Interview with Nurse Lillian Morgan.

[14] Interview with Dr A. Law carried out by S. Pitt on 6 January 1993.

[15] Interview with Dr Baker carried out by S. Pitt on 5 November 1992.

[16] Young, M. and Willmott, P. (1973), *The Symmetrical Family: A Study of Work and Leisure in the London Region* (London, Routledge and Kegan Paul), p. 93.

[17] Interview with Sister Hughes carried out by S. Pitt on 20 October 1992.

[18] Interview with Nurse Janey Jones.

[19] Interview with Sister Gerty Morgan.

[20] Interview with Sister Howell carried out by S. Pitt on 23 October 1992.

[21] Interview with Sister Hughes.

[22] Interview with Dr A. Law.

[23] Interview with Dr W. O. Williams carried out by S. Pitt on 25 September 1992.

[24] Myles, M. F. (1953), *A Textbook for Midwives* (Edinburgh and London, E. & S. Livingstone), p. 284.

[25] Thomas, F. D. (1953), *Mayes' Handbook for Midwives and Maternity Nurses* (London, Bailliere, Tindall and Cox), pp. 163–7.

[26] See below.

[27] Bailey, R. E. (1972), *Mayes' Midwifery: A Textbook for Midwives* (London, Bailliere Tindall), p. 249.

[28] Clayton, S. G., Fraser, D. and Lewis, T. L. T. (eds) (1972), *Obstetrics by Ten Teachers* (London, Edward Arnold), p. 492.

[29] Tew, M. (1990) *Safer Childbirth? A Critical History of Maternity Care* (London, Chapman and Hall), p. 101.

[30] Oakley, A. (1984), *The Captured Womb: A History of the Medical Care of Pregnant Women* (Oxford, Blackwell), p. 182.

[31] Petchesky, R. P. (1987), 'Foetal images: the power of visual culture in the politics of reproduction', in Stanworth, M. (ed.), *Reproductive Technologies: Gender, Motherhood and Medicine* (Cambridge, Polity Press), pp. 57–80 (58–63).

[32] Ibid., p. 65.

[33] Myles, *A Textbook for Midwives*, pp. 117–18.

[34] Clayton, Fraser and Lewis, *Obstetrics*, p. 135.

[35] Jordanova, L. (1989) *Sexual Visions: Images of Gender in Science and Medicine between the Eighteenth and Twentieth Centuries* (London, Harvester Wheatsheaf), p. 45.

[36] Tew, *Safer Childbirth?*, p. 43.

[37] Clayton, Fraser and Lewis, *Obstetrics*, p. 132.

9

'It's a Funny Job Really': The Contradictions of Health Visiting

ᥤ

ANTHEA SYMONDS

Introduction

This chapter has two main purposes: firstly, to uncover the contradictions and ambiguities inherent in health visiting; and secondly, to reveal the responses and strategies employed by a set of health visitors in their everyday practice. The site of the study was an area of south Wales, on the M4 corridor, which although covered by one local trust, nevertheless contained localities which were socially and economically diverse. The focus will be upon two main areas of health visiting: the site and organization of practice; and its stated objective and purpose, both of which form an occupational identity. Within each of these areas health visitors engage in a set of strategies and negotiations by which they attempt to define their own occupational purpose and identity. In order to understand fully the situation in which the health visitors in this study were placed, a brief historical review of the policies, which sited health visiting in a primary health-care setting, and the definition of professional practice and objectives, will set the scene. This study must also be placed within a definition of health visiting as a gendered practice and occupation. This is an essential ingredient both to the study and to an understanding of the professional and political debates surrounding the future of health visiting. How can health visiting be understood as a gendered practice?

'Women's Work in a Man's World'

This is how Celia Davies[1] has described the organization, practice and definition of health visiting. I wish to utilize her definition of gender relations in health visiting to mean primarily a cultural practice. In terms of its status within the health service, health visiting, like nursing, can be defined as a feminized 'semi-profession' which Anne Witz[2] and Jeff Hearn[3] have described and analysed. This term denotes a female-dominated occupation (such as nursing, midwifery and radiography) which exists as an intermediary between the dominant masculinized medical profession and the population.

But, historically, health visiting has also been placed as an intermediary between the masculinized organization of public health and a predominantly female client group. As Celia Davies has chronicled, the origin of health visiting in the nineteenth century was within the sphere of public health, but, as women, health visitors were consigned to work in the private sphere of the home with mothers and children.[4] Men, on the other hand, filled the posts of public (later environmental) health inspectors exercising authority in the public sphere.

Masculinity and femininity existed therefore as cultural divisions of practice which were embodied in the persons of men and women who were designated to separate activities and responsibilities. Both public health and medicine were defined within a 'masculine' school of values based upon 'command and control'.[5] This emphasis also included a belief in scientific objectivity and neutrality which invalidated empathetic or emotional interaction. Health visiting which operated within this sphere therefore occupied a contradictory and peripheral position based upon a different set of values which emphasized support and trust. This division is of great significance when analysing the value placed upon the perceived purpose of practice.

As writers on the nineteenth-century development of health visiting, such as Davin[6] and Symonds,[7] have noted, the objective of their practice was the education of working-class women in mothering skills and the reinforcement of the private sphere of the home as the basis of female identity. This practice took place within a masculine paradigm of work and authority structures but was based upon the 'policing' of other women. Therefore, health visiting often did not appear as 'real work', and because of its private nature it remained peripheral to the mainstream provision of health care. This opacity of purpose and practice has prompted some sociological research into the 'real' or actual practice of health visitors. Studies have described the way in which health visitors engage in 'fringe' work[8] and shown that much of everyday health visiting involving the strengthening of networks of support, giving help in a variety of circumstances and generally 'being there' for vulnerable women and children, is officially unrecorded and therefore undervalued. As we shall see, the relationship between the health visitor, as a woman representing an authority structure, and the mothers, with whom she may empathize, but who are the objects of practice, can be a contradictory one. As women, many of the health visitors in the study were 'on the side' of the women they were employed to exercise a degree of control over. This was especially true of those who came from the same area and shared many of the cultural values and attitudes of the women themselves.

The following study illustrates the responses of health visitors to the constraints of an organizational structure and the imposition by that structure of objectives which effectively marginalize the 'real' meaning of their practice.

Background to the Study

The following observations were the result of a four-month study of health visiting practice in a community trust area of south Wales during the summer and autumn of 1996. This was essentially an observational exercise, during which I accompanied twenty-seven health visitors on their daily rounds, attended baby clinics in both community health centres and GP practices, 'sat in' on antenatal interviews and sex advice clinics, watched innumerable child development tests, and talked to health visitors about their practice and how they perceived its purpose and meaning. I also attended some management meetings with both staff and potential GP contractors. I recorded some of the interviews, others I scribbled down in my field notes during the course of the day. The area, which was covered by the trust, was a mixed one, comprising five zones of health visiting practice:

(a) an old colliery town and surrounding estates and villages which contained a high percentage of deprivation and unemployment and had a high rate of young single mothers (six health visitors);

(b) affluent commuter villages and a wealthy retirement area but which also contained an RAF camp, which was shortly to close (five health visitors);

(c) a traditional Valleys area with a high proportion of elderly people, unemployment, extended families and single mothers (four health visitors);

(d) a large urban area and surrounding villages which contained a vast housing estate that was predominantly privately owned but also contained a small area of housing association houses (eight health visitors);

(e) a seaside town which was a mixture of large and affluent houses, retirement bungalows and caravan sites but with evidence of urban decline and deprivation. The population was a mixture of local permanent residents and seasonal workers (four health visitors).

In the colliery town and surrounding areas, the Valleys (a and c), and in one section of the urban area (d), the health visitor still worked semi-autonomously from the local community clinic. The significance of this will become clear in the description of the historical changes to health visiting which are described in the following section. In the areas where a community involvement still remained, their 'attachment' to local GP practices involved attending a weekly baby clinic in the surgery and receiving referrals by phone or by going to the practice to 'pick up'. In contrast, the health visitors in the other areas were sited in the GP practices in widely divergent conditions which ranged from a damp and mildewed basement to the purpose-built 'fund-holder' pine and formica office (areas d and e). All shared their premises with other community nurses and services including community dentists, chiropodists, school nurses and audiologists. Well-baby clinics in all areas continued to be held in community clinics in the centre of the town, on the housing estate or local villages, as well as in the local practice, although during the period of the research one community clinic (in one Valley area) was closed by the local community trust. All the health visitors I accompanied worked full-time, and all were women, as were the other community-based personnel. The majority of their work concentrated on mothers and children in various settings. There were 'special referrals' for a minority of other visits with elderly or disabled people.

This project was essentially one of exploration; it does not claim to be of a generalist or universal application. There may be specifically regional and cultural aspects which are not to be found elsewhere, but it did reveal some of the cultural and organizational structures and contradictions which health visitors were experiencing and the ways in which these were the subject of adherence, negotiation or resistance by them.

The Site of Health Visiting, Public Health and General Practice

A recognition of the changing geographical site of health visiting from its nineteenth-century roots through to the present is crucial to an understanding of the contradictions experienced by health visitors in their practice. The origins of health visiting lie within the sphere and philosophy of public health. But it must be emphasized that this sphere was as much a geographical setting as an organizational description. As Dingwall[9] illustrates, throughout the transition of health visiting from a service organized by philanthropic societies to its 'take-up' by the state, the site of practice was that of the locality or neighbourhood. In the early years of the twentieth century, local authorities, under the supervision of medical officers of health, employed health visitors and their services were delivered to whole neighbourhoods. This concentration upon a geographical area and its inhabitants became known as the 'patch system'. Because the predominant objective of health visiting was the education of working-class mothers in areas of high infant mortality, it was inevitable that the service would be concentrated upon areas of poverty and deprivation. However, health visiting was a universalist service offered to all the target population and did not carry the stigma attached to the recipients of social-work services.

The Maternal and Child Welfare Act of 1918 led to the construction of local authority community clinics as the public site of health visiting practice. After the Second World War, the foundation of the National Health Service made health visiting a statutory universalist service to be provided by all county councils and boroughs. Although the 1950s placed health visiting as an occupation firmly within the boundaries of the health service and nursing, its geographical site of practice remained that of the locality or neighbourhood. This structure was reinforced by the recommendations of the Jameson Report[10] which set out the ratios of health visitors to size of local population.

The NHS (Reorganization) Act of 1974 radically changed the geographical site of the service by moving the employment of health visitors from local authorities to area health authorities and to a system of 'attachment' to individual GP practices. On reflection, this move can be seen to highlight the underlying ambiguity of the role and purpose of health visiting. Many GPs were totally ignorant of the function of health visiting as it had previously existed in the separate sphere of public health and local authority organization. But as Robert Dingwall records, the dominant assumption among doctors and other practice staff was that health visitors were 'mere auxiliaries whose work would be strictly under the GPs control'.[11] By 1982, it was calculated that 80 per cent of health visitors were attached to general practices,[12] and the inherent ambiguity of their location was to become apparent as the organization of general practice itself became the target of policy changes.

General practice was the focus of two major changes during the 1980s and early 1990s; firstly, the imposition of the new GP contract with its emphasis on health education and the payment for the achievement of pre-set health gain targets (including immunization and child surveillance) which were set out in the White Paper *Promoting Better Health*.[13] This meant that the weekly baby clinics became increasingly sited at the GP surgery rather than in the community-based clinic. The significance of this change for health visitors is described in the following section. Secondly, the advent of fund-holding and the creation of the internal market in health care which were set in motion by the White Paper *Working for Patients*,[14] were to have a profound effect on the perception of the function of the service. Both of these developments changed the organization and, I would argue, the culture of general practice, and rendered the position of health visitors within this site even more ambiguous. The identification of the fund-holding GP as the 'purchaser' of health visiting services via contracts entered into with community health trusts, health authorities and other organizations was implemented by the NHS and Community Care Act in 1990.

The Health Visitor Association (HVA), the representative organization of health visitors, was largely opposed to most of these measures, and this opposition was articulated via the journal, *Health Visitor*. One of the areas of concern was that GPs would prefer to use practice nurses (who were employed directly by them) to undertake work previously the province of health visitors.[15] The fear that GPs would therefore not 'purchase' the services of health visitors at all, thus calling into question the future existence of the service, prompted the HVA to call for a mass lobby of Parliament to protest against the measures.[16] But despite this profession-based opposition, government policies were further to extend fund-holding and to place health visiting in a position of having to 'market' the service to the prospective purchasers.

This development prompted a professional concern with the future of public health in a wider sense. A guidance document for fund-holders[17] was published which outlined the extent of 'flexibility' allowed to GPs in the setting of health visitors' work, including the allocation of a vague 'notional' amount of time to be set aside for 'public health', but this did not really allay the fears of the profession.[18] The next development was the move to integrate health visitors into all primary health-care GP-led 'teams' and to place them under the direct management of the practice.[19] Many in the profession felt that this development would finally eradicate any claim that health visiting was an autonomous profession, and would make health visitors 'isolated and vulnerable'.[20] The prospect of direct employment by individual practices was finally spelled out in the White Paper *Choice and Opportunity: Primary Health Care – The Future*, published at the end of 1996.[21] This is the framework surrounding the research study which I began in late 1996. The health visitors with whom I worked were affected by all the policy shifts, job insecurity and a lack of self-confidence in their own worth which had resulted from the upheavals of the preceding years. The following account of the responses and strategies employed by some health visitors mostly working within the orbit of general practice and its power relations must be placed against this background.

Site, Territory and Power Relations

The significance of the siting of health visiting within a general
practice was perceived in varying degrees in different areas. In the
areas where health visiting had not yet been sited in a practice,
there was a strongly articulated opposition to the development. For
instance, in the Valleys area, a health visitor stated: 'there has
always been a patch system here, it's traditional really' and went on
to claim: 'The day we move into a GP's surgery is the day I leave.' In
the other area where the health visitors still worked from the
community clinic (area a), the trust management was seeking to
move them to a different location, disused shop premises in the
high street, but not to place them in the GP's practice. The health
visitors there were also predominantly 'negative' about the siting of
health visitors actually in the practice premises. 'There are pros
and cons (to moving into GP practice) but I think it's better to be
separate, GPs know where we are and can always contact us'
(health visitor in colliery town).

Conversely, a health visitor working from new GP practice
premises on a large urban estate welcomed the clear identity which
the situation gave her: 'I feel that we are seen as a part of the primary
health care team, people know where we are and what our place is.'
It was, however, the relationship with the GP that health visitors
regarded as of primary importance, irrespective of geographical
proximity. Interestingly, all claimed a 'close working relationship'
with the GPs. But the nature of this relationship was not clearly
defined and remained ambiguous. A Valleys-based health visitor,
despite her opposition to the move into a practice, insisted: 'we
have a good relationship with GPs – they're always on the phone.'
But an alternative interpretation was gained when, on one
occasion, a health visitor who wished to see a doctor after a baby
clinic in the surgery, was forced to wait outside the door until, as
she put it, 'I can just nip in before the next patient'. This was very
reminiscent of a similar working situation described by Dingwall[22]
over twenty years previously.

Even when health visitors were working on the site of the
practice surgery itself, the closeness of the relationship was difficult to perceive. This can be illustrated by the example of a health
visitor who was very enthusiastic about being in a new GP fund-
holding practice and said: 'We are in closer contact here. I feel that

they know me better here and know what I do.' She then led me to 'her' office, which had 'Health Visitor' on the door but which she shared with the community nurse, a part-time pharmacist and a counsellor. She then introduced me to the senior partner of the practice and the following encounter took place.

> Health Visitor: Oh, doctor – this is Dr Anthea Symonds, she's here doing some research on health visiting.
> Doctor: Oh and what are you looking at specifically?
> Researcher: I'm going around with health visitors to see just what they do and how they practise.
> Doctor: When you find out, let me know. I've often wondered.
> [Nervous laughter all round.]

In another area, the three health visitors were all enthusiastic about their purpose-built office in a new surgery, where they all claimed, 'we have great co-operation with GPs now'. I did not, however, observe one personal contact between them and any of the five GPs in two weeks.

The legitimacy of the authority of the GP to control the sphere of their working practice was widely accepted, even if the day-to-day constraint was sometimes resented. One health visitor working with women in the local refuge but based in a fund-holding practice in a large urban centre reported: 'The GPs don't like it. They said that they would be high demand patients – you know what they're like.' Nevertheless, this particular health visitor had continued to work with the refuge, stating defiantly of the GPs: 'They don't employ me, but they seem to think that they do.'

A similar conflict arose with the setting up of a community house on a new estate funded by the National Children's Homes, the housing association and local social services. Health visitors were to set up a weekly rota system of attendance at a 'drop-in' morning. I attended a meeting of health visitors to discuss the project and though all were enthusiastic about the idea they articulated concerns about the attitude of 'their' GPs.

> Health Visitor 1: The GPs won't be keen as I don't have any families on that estate.
> Health Visitor 2: That's always a worry with GPs isn't it? Ours are not keen at all.

> Health Visitor 3: I don't mind taking a turn but GPs won't be keen, we don't do that estate.
> Researcher: Are GPs always so territorial?
> Health visitor 1: Yes, but it's got worse since they went fund-holding.

In these instances it was the 'approval' of the GP which was being withheld rather than a total opposition, but nevertheless the power lines were very clearly drawn and the autonomy of these health visitors to work even for a 'notional' percentage of time in public health outside the practice areas was seemingly reduced.

What of the relationship with other members of the 'team' in the practice? Even in those practices where the health visitors had their own offices, a degree of marginalization took place, often between them and the practice staff. Offices are frequently shared between health visitors and community nurses. In one area there was only one phone line for the health visitors, nurses, community dentist, chiropodist and speech therapist. In another area, the practice manager prohibited health visitors' use of the car park, which necessitated them carrying equipment from the street. But there was one site where the ambiguities of the role of health visitor within the medically dominated setting were particularly marked: the weekly well-baby clinic.

The Practice-Based Clinic: A Contested Territory

In the setting of the GP surgery, the clinics take place in the afternoons when the 'normal' business of the practice is suspended. This has the effect of setting up a disjuncture between the surgery setting, the rows of chairs, medical and health promotion posters, reception desk, and the 'special' nature of the subjects of attention: women, babies and young children. In one such practice, the receptionist greeted the arrival of the health visitors with the cry, 'Oh God! it's screaming kids' day.' The bureaucratic nature of the 'normal' surgery, however, still persists. People's names are taken on entry, babies are weighed in turn, adults sit in the rows of chairs, questions are asked and two sets of record books are examined and filled in. As one health visitor claimed, 'We are obsessed with measuring everything, especially weight. We write it down three times – waste of time and energy.'

One practice had implemented an almost Fordist-type production line. My field notes describe it thus:

> Very hot day. Baby clinic at the top of the building, only window is in roof, very stuffy and airless. Entry to clinic is through a back door at the side where a bell has to be pushed and receptionists in main building automatically release door, and then people have to climb two flights of stairs. On entry into room, people have to take a 'number' from a box. The clinic begins at 2.00 but by 1.45 the room is nearly full. The proceedings are then dominated by 'waiting for doctor' – who arrives at 2.30.
> Health Visitor: 'He's always late, but when he does arrive he goes through them very quickly.'
> Either the practice nurse or the doctor kept coming into room with sheaf of notes and calling numbers. When people had seen the doctor they left via the flight of stairs. The health visitor flitted around the room attempting to talk to people but the constant interruptions and the cramped space made this almost impossible. Practice nurse weighed the babies in a dark corner of the room.

In all the surgery-based clinics, the health visitor is required to fight for a space – geographical and professional: both become contested sites.

In one practice where the health visitors were not directly 'attached' but just attended for the weekly baby clinic, the antagonism was palpable. The health visitor was allotted the nurses' room for a preliminary antenatal consultation (these are often scheduled concurrently with baby clinics), and my field notes recorded the setting.

> No privacy. The room has 2 doors, nurses keep coming backwards and forwards through the room, never knock. The phone rings, a nurse comes in and answers, holds conversation talking across health visitor and young woman. The toilet is also in the room, women enter room to use toilet to give sample. Private conversation impossible. Health visitor looks at me and raises eyes.

In most of the clinics, the practice nurses undertook the weighing of babies but this was frequently done with the health visitor very close by. One health visitor confided to me: 'Quite honestly I wouldn't let them even weigh them. They don't know what to look for, they don't know anything about children.' Health visitors adopted differing techniques in consultations. 'There are two ways of doing it – you either tell them the bare minimum or start on twenty questions.' But at all times within this setting it was necessary for the health visitor to initiate the contact. It was an essentially proactive stance which had to be taken; they had to carve out their own space. One way in which some health visitors attempted to exclude the practice nurses was by addressing every person who entered the room by name and then asking after the baby – also by name. One such greeting I recorded: 'Hello there. How's my beautiful boy today then? Dylan's coming on really well isn't he? Any news on the job? How's the decorating going?' Sometimes they asked questions about other family members to demonstrate their familiarity, this effectively leaving the practice nurse 'outside' the consultation circle. In all the GP surgeries, this model of organization is present to a degree. The surgery 'belongs' to the doctor and practice staff, it is their space. It is a space which is normally concerned with processing illness and is unaccustomed to seeing the healthy. It is run on the value of efficiency, which is defined as speed of throughput, as illustrated by the doctor, who although continually late, 'goes through them'.

The objective of the clinic is also narrowly defined. In two of the clinics people were informed that they must not consult the doctor with any other health problems, but that these must be the subject of a separate appointment. Deviation from strict production targets was not allowed and in fact was termed 'time wasting' by one practice nurse. As has been illustrated, the clinic on the site of the practice was frequently a contested one, with health visitors often occupying the role of an outsider. This may be contrasted with the community clinic-based ones which all the health visitors in the study said that they preferred.

Community Clinics: Home Territory

The community site, unlike that of the surgery, reveals clearly the social and economic composition of the area. It is almost as if the uniformity of the surgery surroundings camouflage social difference, so that a surgery in an area of high deprivation will not appear markedly different from one in a more affluent area.

The buildings in which these clinics took place varied. They included a community hall, an old 1920s maternal welfare clinic, an old miners' welfare hall, a new community centre on an estate and a sports hall on an RAF camp, but they all were a part and reflection of the local communities. Here is an extract from my field notes on a visit to a clinic in a community hall in a small ex-mining village.

> The hall is wooden and has small car park and flowerbeds in front. It is 9.15 and already there are three women sitting on the steps outside with four small children and two pushchairs. Two of the women are smoking. It is a warm day, they smile and nod.
>
> Inside the hall, there are two health visitors there setting up and a young woman who turns out to be the clinic nurse, another young woman comes in with a baby in a 'Moses basket', she is introduced to me as the doctor. The walls contain photographs of events, the pensioners' Christmas lunch, a recent 80th birthday party. There is a small kitchen and the hatch is opened up to reveal a middle-aged woman who is setting out boxes of milk. The kettle is on, and everyone goes in to the kitchen for coffee. The doctor shows photos of the baby, this is her first day back after maternity leave. The 'milk lady' has holiday photos of her recent visit to her daughter in Arizona. The atmosphere is relaxed and friendly. A health visitor explains to me: 'Officially the clinic is from 9.30 to 11.30 but you find that they come in two batches, early and late. You see the benefit pays out at about 11.30 so they either come on their way in or after. We never really finish here until after 12, it has been much later if they all decide to come late.'

This prediction was entirely accurate, and so the lull in the middle of the morning allowed the health visitors to 'catch up' on the paper work and have another cup of coffee, this accompanied by biscuits which the doctor has made.

A health visitor tells me: 'One thing you'll notice in an area like this is the way they dress the babies up. All frills and satin and always in pink or white. They're like little pets really, still it's all they've got.' The clinic is busy. There appears to be a high number of teenage women with babies, accompanied by their mothers, or in four cases by young men. People cluster together in small groups. One young woman came in and asked for a health visitor by name. She was told that she 'was busy but would be out in a minute'. She sits and waits. When the health visitor appeared she went up to her, spoke a few brief words and left. The health visitor came to me and showed me a very tightly folded £5 note. 'Look at this, she couldn't fold it much smaller could she? Bless her! Poor dab! I lent it to her last week, she had nothing but I knew she'd give it back, it's pitiful really isn't it?' A woman and her teenage daughter come in with a small baby. The health visitor said to me:

> Now this is a lovely family. The daughter's only 16 but she's a great mother and the baby is really loved by all the family. When she came home from the hospital they had a banner right across the front of the house with balloons.

The grandmother is the only person in the family working, she has a job as a home help. She is worried about the child benefit which she is getting for her daughter and wonders if she can still get it even though the daughter herself is drawing child benefit for her baby. The health visitor reassures her. The clinic finishes at about 12.30, but the health visitors have eaten sandwiches and are ready to go straight to the afternoon's work.

In this and all the community clinics, health visitors were in control of the work process and their time and were able to exercise a degree of autonomy. They filled in the 'official' time of the clinic on their small Psion computers and then the 'official' lunch hour but in reality these were fictional formal entries which did not convey the real work which had taken place. They have not dominated the space of the clinic; it was in the nature of a shared space, with mothers and families able to open up conversations and seek advice and help on many subjects. This pattern was repeated to some degree in all the community-based clinics in different locations. Health visitors often use them to widen their practice into areas that are outside both the medical model of baby clinics and the strictly delineated management-set tasks. It is here that they can engage in 'fringe work', as it was termed by de la Cuesta.[23] In one clinic on a new estate, health visitors organized a baby clothes swap and an unofficial loan of cots and buggies. In another, a health visitor was 'on the look-out' for one young woman.

> I know he's beating her up, and if she comes down here for milk I can see if she's OK. She won't go to the doctor's but she's got to come here for the milk or send one of the kids and then I can check. I can never see her alone at home as he's always there.

The provision of milk in exchange for tokens (for those in receipt of means-tested benefits) is an integral part of the work in all of the community clinics. Health visitors often use the collection of milk to talk to women about feeding and to initiate contacts with families whom 'you never see, they don't keep appointments and are never in'.

The site of the community clinic is where the health visitors are 'at home' in every sense of the phrase. It is where they can extend their practice and autonomy. Ironically, it was this 'homely' atmosphere that was the source of criticism of the service by the medical profession, who traditionally saw it as 'trivial'.[24] Although a doctor is present, they do not control the space. All the community doctors I encountered were young women with small children who merged easily with the informal and flexible nature of the organization in the community clinic.

Organizational Models of Baby Clinics

In all the areas clinics were held in both the community and the practice surgery. Frequently the same parents would attend both (sometimes within a couple of days) and see the same health visitor both times. By attending the two sites in the same area often within the same week, I was able to construct the following comparative model: the 'practice-based' model and the 'community-based' model. The weekly well-baby clinic is the anchor of health visiting, it is the one site where health visitors are visible to all, available and accessible. It is also a *public* site as opposed to the *private* sphere of home visiting. But the 'public' nature of the practice-based clinic was circumscribed by the restriction of access to patients of the practice only. This meant the curtailment of health visitor involvement in areas of social concern external to narrowly defined health issues, and the imposition of a bureaucratic discipline upon the interaction between health visitors and mothers. Conversely, the 'community-based' model operating in the community clinics allowed for a wider involvement by the health visitor in other areas of social care and also gave more space to mothers. The significance of the division between the two settings is illustrated in Tables 9.1 and 9.2:

Table 9.1 Practice-based model

Organizational structure	Bureaucratic
Site	GP surgery 'out of hours'
Space	Doctor/practice nurse-dominated
Subject	Mothers and babies as 'patients'
Authority	Bureaucratic hierarchical
Other services	None
Role of HV	Marginalized

Table 9.2 Community-based model

Organizational structure	Loose and open
Site	Community clinic
Space	Health visitor facilitated
Subject	Mothers and babies as clients/extended family
Authority	Consultative
Other services	Sales of milk/exchange of tokens, baby clothes 'swap', social networking
Role of HV	Central

Interestingly, a previous study of the two types of clinic[25] defined the different structures they observed as the 'paediatric' and the 'welfare' models. This division between a medical model and a social model of care is still apparent and involves not only a different authority structure but also a different culture. The looser structure of the community clinic meant that health visitors could adapt to the needs and demands of the wider community. As one health visitor said: 'The GPs don't like the community clinics much as it can mean that we can spend time with people who are not patients of the practice but in the surgery they can check.' The necessity to adjust to the expectations and needs of the client group is illustrated by the way in which health visitors adopt a strategy of adaptation within the officially designated objective and purpose of their practice.

Health Visiting: Its Objective and Purpose

Historically, the objective and purpose of health visiting has been inextricably linked not only to nursing, but also to education, social work, and the now defunct hospital almoner service. The boundaries between the occupations often appeared blurred despite moves by the professional body of health visitors to clarify its position concretely as a distinct occupation. Although originally health visitors did not have to be nurses, access to health visiting had required a post-nursing course of training and a midwifery qualification since the inter-war years, and this route was firmly established within the NHS after 1948. However, it was the educative function of health visiting and its focus upon the 'healthy' rather than the 'sick' population which had always distinguished it from nursing. As Jane Robinson has noted, within this setting health visiting was 'beset with problems of role identity'.[26] It could also be argued that yet another ambiguity of purpose is revealed by this specific function of education as it placed health visiting in a 'policing' rather than a primarily 'caring' role.[27]

The expansion of the state social services in the post-war period meant that health visiting practice, by now undertaken by qualified nurses, required official clarification of purpose to distinguish it from the expanding profession of social work. The Jameson Report in 1956[28] set out the area of practice to encompass: child guidance, the care of handicapped people at home, health education, the visiting of frail elderly and disabled people and the follow-up of discharged patients (taking this responsibility from the hospital almoner service). This placed the remit of health visiting firmly within the boundaries of the health service and separated from social work.[29] In 1962, the two occupations were to be formally divided when the respective responsibility for social work and health visiting training came under the sphere of the Council for Education and Training in Social Work (CCETSW) and the Council for Education and Training of Health Visitors (CETHV). However, the links between them were not entirely broken as the two bodies were responsible for placing the acquisition of the qualifying diplomas for both health visiting and social work within higher education. Interestingly, the curriculum for the health visiting diploma included a grounding in 'the social as well as the medical sciences',[30] which once again illustrated a blurring of the boundaries between the 'social' and 'health' orientation of health visiting practice.

Following the restructuring after 1974 and the closer attachment to the site of medical practice, the CETHV was prompted to set out clearly the four basic principles of health visiting. These were: the search for health needs, the stimulation of awareness of need, the influence on policies affecting health and the facilitation of health-enhancing activities.[31] This amalgamation of health care, education, social awareness and support still forms the basis of the identity of health visiting as a distinctive practice from nursing. However, the separate professional organization of health visiting ended with the demise of the CETHV in 1982 and its replacement by the United Kingdom Central Council for Nursing, Midwifery and Health Visiting (UKCC). In many ways this move could be seen as a reflection of the absorption of health visiting into the primary health-care 'team' based in the GP practice.

The organizational and philosophical changes within the health service during the 1980s were to pose a problem for the 'reality' of health visiting practice. The adoption by a cost-conscious general management of 'objective' criteria of effectiveness of the service was often translated into a 'checklist ticking approach'[32] to practice. The evaluative criteria imposed by many managers (including the trust where the study was based) included the counting of numbers of contacts made and the setting of statutory health gain targets. This attempt to validate health visiting practice 'scientifically' had the effect of narrowing its purpose from that set out in the four basic principles. In effect, the social-care element was eradicated and the educative function reduced to the giving of official health 'messages'. Many of the health visitors I worked with experienced a contradiction between the achievement of the formally set objectives and the maintenance of their socially supportive relationship with mothers and families.

Negotiating the 'Message'

Under the constant pressure to 'prove' effectiveness in order to 'sell' the services of health visitors to purchasers, the trust management instituted a list of health-education targets to be achieved. These involved the usual advice on diet, weaning and smoking, and encouragement to breast-feed with recommended 'targets' to be reached. There was a marked difference in methods of implementation of this advice between those working in socially deprived compared with more affluent areas.

For many health visitors working with women and families living in deprived conditions, the giving of such 'lifestyle' advice was often seen as both contentious and counterproductive. As one health visitor said: 'I can see by the look in their eyes that if I start on healthy eating and all that stuff, I've lost them.' Another said:

> We are supposed to give diet advice to elderly people when we visit – I think it's insulting. After all if they've survived until eighty after all they've been through all their lives what the hell does it matter what they eat? It can't have done them much harm, can it?

Another said: 'There's far too much fuss about healthy eating and all that, it gets on peoples' nerves – I don't do it.' Another made the point:

> You notice it's all anti-smoking. They don't go on so much about drink do they? That's because they [managers – my emphasis] all drink. I don't agree with the anti-smoking policy in hospitals. A lot of elderly people round here won't go in because of it.

It was noticeable that many health visitors negotiated this contradictory role by distancing themselves from the advice they were contracted to give. The method most adopted was to put themselves in the role of a messenger, in the following ways:

> You know that we've got to tell you that smoking is no good for you – and it isn't – but I know it's hard: just try to cut down to five a day.

> Well I'm not going to go on at you, but it's the policy.

> I have to tell you this – but I must admit I enjoy my chips too.

In the affluent commuter village, however, the problem of delivering the 'message' was of a different order. Here, health visitors often felt rather intimidated by the middle-class and educated mothers, some of whom were doctors themselves or doctors' wives, especially those who were seen as 'knowing everything – they tell you'. As one said to me after a home visit to one such family:

> Can you imagine telling her about diet and all that, she knows more than I do. I did say to her about the new advice on when to start them on solids and she gave me a load of stuff about some research in Australia which disproved the Coma research.

One health visitor who had previously worked in the adjacent
socially deprived area said:

> We are seen as a threat in places like ———. They don't want us telling
> them what to eat and giving advice – they just want us to clear off – but
> here they get worried about things that the others don't even know
> exist!
>   In an area like this, you can do as much or as little as you want to do.
> They don't need a lot of the advice we're supposed to give but they do
> have problems, they get uptight about things that others wouldn't think
> twice about – like do they play with their children enough?

In this educative role, health visitors often 'negotiated' with the
transmission of messages, adapting to the social reality of their
client group. This strategy, which de la Cuesta[33] has termed 'negotiation' and 'compromise', is entered into both as a means of resistance to management directives and also as a means of 'selling'
themselves to a client group. This strategy of adaptation illustrates
both an awareness of the limitations of a management directive
approach and recognition of the necessity of gaining what Abbot
and Sapsford[34] have called 'acceptance' by clients.

'It's a funny job really'

Health visitors themselves articulated many of the concerns over
the purpose of health visiting as practised in the current organizational structure and reflected on the contradictions within which
they worked.

> Health visiting is just a dumping ground. Every time they think of
> something and don't know who to get to do it, they land it on us.

> We're just a jack of all trades. What makes me sick is that we have to
> creep to the bloody doctors all the time.

> It's a funny job really, I often wonder what are we really doing and what
> do we achieve?

> We should be with social workers, they're our natural allies.

The area which many perceived as their strength and identity was
the possession of a knowledge of social reality as opposed to the

unreality exhibited by both managers and doctors. As one health visitor reported:

> I went to a meeting the other week and this jumped-up health-education or promotion manager, he was on about healthy eating. A lot of us were getting fed up and angry and then he said 'Why don't people eat properly?', and one of us said 'poverty'. He said 'I knew you were going to say that but it isn't true, they need life-skills' I ask you! What planet do they live on?

This extract sums up the belief held by many health visitors that they possess knowledge and experience of the 'real world' as opposed to the ignorance of managers and GPs. The idea that there is a world inhabited by themselves and their client group to which those in authority do not have access is a source of identity and a means of resistance. Another health visitor in recounting a meeting with a manager said:

> There was this one on about information technology and he said, 'By the year 2000 everyone will be on the internet, it will be in everyone's home and they will be communicating with Australia just as you talk to people next door.' I go to places where a lot of them haven't even got a phone! They want to get in the real world.

One health visitor used this means to state her objection to the moving of the baby clinics to the local surgery: 'GPs don't seem to realize that a lot of women just can't get to clinics in town. They don't have a car and the bus journey is horrendous with small kids. They haven't got a clue.'

I have used these extracts to pinpoint a response to a contradiction experienced by many in health visiting. This involves the recognition of a solidarity with 'their' area and the lives of other women and at the same time an acknowledgement of their own subordinated position within the organizational structure.

Conclusion

I have argued that the current practice of health visiting is determined by many factors, including spatial territory and constructed power relations, ambiguity of identity and purpose, and an organizational structure within which it is marginalized. The principal problem in searching for a definition of health visiting is its occupational place at the intersection between health and social care. As policies and institutional structures, which followed from the increase in state intervention in the twentieth century, increasingly separated these two spheres, so the ambiguous position of health visiting was highlighted. Although brought into the sphere of the health service, composed of trained nurses and placed within a GP practice base, health visiting never really 'fitted'. Health visiting has always been placed within a set of contradictions involving the public and private sphere of activity and power relations. The practice of health visiting has also, as Jane Robinson[35] has argued, faced the 'double bind' of existing within both collective and individual health care. This 'split' existence rendered health visiting vulnerable when the service was subjected to systems of evaluation and cost-effectiveness within the confines of a medically driven organizational structure. This structure was based on a narrow definition of health and health care, and required health visitors to restrict their practice to a predetermined set of 'targets' and activities. Every day, in their 'normal' practice, health visitors live these contradictions. But they also construct responses of accommodation and strategies of resistance in order to make sense of the reality of their practice. But these responses are essentially reactive ones, which pinpoint their position as a feminized semi-profession.

The identity of the occupation, however, remains as problematic as ever and the distinction between health and social care in the implementation of community-based care has further highlighted the ambiguities. Interestingly, the advent of community care policies and the development of a child protection service has increasingly meant that health visitors have become more involved with social workers in case conferences and meetings. The barriers between the purpose of the two occupations have become more blurred. But, at the same time, the changing imperatives placed upon GP practices have meant that the medicalization of child health has tied the health visitor more closely to the 'nursing' aspect.

But what of the future direction of health visiting? In 1999 the government issued its consultation document, *Supporting Families*, which particularly highlighted an 'enhanced role for health visitors'.[36] In this, it was specifically stated that health visiting should be expanded to incorporate work actively to prevent social exclusion and family breakdown, and increased funding for a newly constituted service was promised. In Wales, where historically there has always been great political support for public health issues, the White Paper, *Better Health – Better Wales*,[37] pinpointed health visitors as key providers of a proactive service to children and young people as well as to other disadvantaged groups. In December 1999 the National Assembly for Wales commissioned a review of health visiting and school nursing services in order to plan for future demand. Current projects under the Sure Start programme appear to utilize health visitors as key partners. It would appear then that health visiting is on the brink of a revival in its role in public health and community development. Many of the health visitors with whom I worked were already individually actively involved in this role, even though they had been placed in an organizational setting during the 1980s and 1990s which was often antagonistic to these aims and objectives. The contradictions between public and private, collective and individual delivery of health care and between a market and a public-service approach, which lie at the heart of health visiting, still remain to be solved. Meanwhile, health visitors themselves live these contradictions in their daily practice.

Notes

[1] Davies, C. (1997), 'Health visiting: women's work in a man's world', *Health Visitor*, 70, 110–11.

[2] Witz, A. (1992), *Professions and Patriarchy* (London, Routledge).

[3] Hearn, J. (1982), 'Notes on patriarchy, professionalisation and the semi-professions', *Sociology*, 16.

[4] Davies, C. (1998), 'The health visitor as mother's friend', *Social History of Medicine* 1, 39–59.

[5] Davies, 'Health visiting', 111.

[6] Davin, A. (1978), 'Imperialism and motherhood', *History Workshop*, 5, 9–65.

[7] Symonds, A. (1991), 'Angels and interfering busybodies: a social construction of two occupations', *Sociology of Health and Illness*, 13, 249–64.

[8] De la Cuesta, C. (1993), 'Fringe work: peripheral work in health visiting', *Sociology of Health and Illness*, 15, 665–81.

[9] Dingwall, R. (1977), 'Collectivism, regionalism and feminism: health visiting and British social policy 1850–1975', *Journal of Social Policy*, 6, 291–315.

[10] Ministry of Health (1956), *An Inquiry into Health Visiting: Report of a Working Party of the field of Work,Training and Recruitment of Health Visitors* (Jameson Report) (London, HMSO).

[11] Dingwall, R. (1977), *The Social Organization of Health Visitor Training* (London, Croom Helm), p. 143.

[12] Office of Population Censuses and Surveys (1982), *Nurses Working in the Community* (London, HMSO).

[13] Department of Health (1987), *Promoting Better Health* (London, HMSO).

[14] Department of Health (1989), *Working for Patients* (London, HMSO).

[15] Potrykus, C. (1989), 'Facing the challenge of GP contracts', *Health Visitor*, 62, 363–4.

[16] Jackson, C. (1990), 'Pulling the plug on the NHS', *Health Visitor*, 63, 43–5.

[17] National Health Service Management Executive (NHSME) (1992), *Guidance on the Extension of the Hospital and Community Health Services Elements of GP Fund-holding Scheme from April 1993* (London, NHSME).

[18] Potrykus, C. (1992), 'Guidance a "Mixed Blessing"', *Health Visitor*, 65, 300–2.

[19] NHSME (1994), *New World, New Opportunities* (London, NHSME).

[20] Jackson, C. (1994), 'New World, New Dilemmas', *Health Visitor*, 67, 8–9.

[21] Department of Health (1996), *Choice and Opportunity: Primary Care – The Future* (London, HMSO).

[22] Dingwall, R. (1974), 'A team role for ancillary staff', *Health and Social Service Journal*, 7 September, 2032–3.

[23] De la Cuesta, 'Fringe work'.

[24] Ibid., 34.

[25] Stacey, M. and Davies, C. (1983), *Division of Labour in Child Health Care: Final Report to SSRC 1983* (Warwick, University of Warwick, Department of Sociology), p. 67.

[26] Robinson, J (1985), 'Health visiting and health', in White, R. (ed.), *Political Issues in Nursing* (London, Wiley).

[27] Dingwall, R. and Robinson, K. (1993), 'Policing the family? Health visiting and the public surveillance of private behaviour', in Beattie, A. (ed.), *Health and Wellbeing: A Reader* (Basingstoke, Macmillan and Open University); Abbott, P. and Sapsford, R. (1990), 'Health visiting: policing the family?', in Abbott, P. and Wallace, C. (eds), *Sociology of the Caring Professions* (Brighton, Falmer Press).

[28] Ministry of Health, *Inquiry into Health Visiting*.

[29] Ibid., p. 160.

[30] Kelly, A., Thome, R. and Mabbett, G. (1998), 'Professions and community nursing', in Symonds, A. and Kelly, A. (eds), *The Social Construction of Community Care* (Basingstoke, Macmillan), p. 160.

[31] CETHV (1977), *Principles of Health Visiting* (London, CETHV).

[32] Goodwin, S. (1988), 'Whither health visiting?', *Health Visitor*, 61, 379–83.

[33] De la Cuesta, C. (1994), 'Marketing: a process in health visiting', *Journal of Advanced Nursing*, 19, 347–53.

[34] Abbott and Sapsford, 'Health visiting'.

[35] Robinson, 'Health visiting and health'.

[36] Home Office (1999), *Supporting Families* (London, HMSO).

[37] Welsh Office (1998), *Better Health – Better Wales* (Cardiff, HMSO).

10

Water, Health and the Public/Private Interface

❧

MARK DRAKEFORD

Introduction

This chapter deals with the supply of one of the most basic house-hold essentials in Wales. Whether organized on a public or private basis it is also, as the Dŵr Cymru Customer Report for 1993–4[1] puts it, one for which 'our customers have no choice but to rely on Dŵr Cymru'. Against that basic background, the chapter aims to draw together two fundamental sets of relationships and to explore the associations between them. The first lies in the connection between water and health; the second in the connection between water, health and the shifting boundary of ownership within the industry. The account which I hope to offer begins with a brief ground-clearing statement of position in relation to both main sets of relationships. The chapter then turns to its more detailed consideration of the impact between ownership and health issues in the water industry in the decade which has followed privatization in 1989. This discussion aims to divide consideration at this point between the policies followed in the remaining years of Conservative administration and the emerging approach of New Labour.

Water and health

The connection between water and health has already been well explored in this book in the chapter by Coopey and Roberts.[2] Their contention that politics and civic pride played an important role in the increasing municipalization of water supply is a significant contribution to our understanding of the development of public provision in this area. It does not, of course, undermine the claims which have been made for public health gains from improved supply: it supplements, rather than supplants such earlier accounts. These remain rooted, as the most recent report of the Chief Medical Officer of Health[3] makes clear, in the belief that public health gains generally in Britain proceeded by expansion from their 'original sanitary base'. Yet, in our own times, the relationship between health and access to a sufficient supply of clean water has been called into question. In order to make clear the perspective adopted in this chapter, therefore, it is as well to begin by repeating the most recent findings of the Global Anti-Incinerator Alliance (GAIA) that, 'an estimated 80 per cent of all diseases and over one third of deaths in developing countries are caused by the consumption of contaminated water, and on average as much as one tenth of each person's productive time is sacrificed to water-related diseases'.[4] Despite the improvements brought about during the 1980s United Nations-sponsored International Drinking Water Supply and Sanitation Decade, one in three people in the developing world still lacks these two most basic requirements for health and dignity. Even when water is available, the cost for poor people can be prohibitive, a fact which finds a striking parallel in the experience of the poorest customers of Britain's privatized utilities today.[5]

In case the suspicion lingers, however, that these connections are important only in far-away places, amongst people who live in very different circumstances, the basic premise upon which the United Nations campaign was based is worth quoting at this point: 'all people, whatever their stage of development and their social and economic conditions, have the right to have access to drinking-water in quantities and of a quality equal to their basic needs.' These concerns are echoed, more locally, in two reports published by the British Medical Association (BMA), which set out the connections between access to clean water and health in the British context. Proceeding from first principles that clean water is an essential public health need and a health right, the first BMA report,[6] nevertheless, drew impetus from 'the dramatic rise in cases of dysentery and hepatitis A in England and Wales [which] has drawn attention to the issue of water disconnection'.

Public debate of the BMA findings was answered by the government of the day with a suggestion that no *causal connection* had been established between a lack of water and the rise in infectious diseases which are associated with a lack of a clean supply. In fact, as the BMA report[7] explained, 'few research studies have attempted to identify a causal link between water disconnections and ill-health'. There are, however, very good reasons for this lack of research, including the wealth of previous evidence of the relationship between the provision of pure, clear water and public health, so that 'it therefore seems irrational to question whether or not water is necessary to prevent the spread of infectious diseases in the late twentieth century'.[8] The same government response, however, was still unveiled in response to the second BMA report in 1996. Replying to the report's call to make disconnection of water illegal because of the risk to public health, the Department of Health issued a statement: 'we have never been able to establish any direct relationship between water disconnection and the spread of communicable diseases in the UK.'[9] Yet, as Middleton and Saunders[10] succinctly put it, 'water is vital to disrupting the chain of person-to-person spread infection; there is no need for a definitive study arising from a grand experiment in social policy. We know that lack of water is bad for public health.' The enduring truth of this basic connection forms one of the central pillars upon which the argument of this chapter is constructed.

Water and ownership

If the basic connection between water and health is one which need not detain us any further, the second main theme of this chapter – the connection between forms of ownership and the water/health nexus – is more controversial. In this section, I set out briefly the changing pattern of ownership which culminated in the privatization of the water industry in England and Wales in 1989, as a prelude to discussion of the health issues which emerged in the years which immediately followed. The chapter of Coopey and Roberts[11] traces the expanding boundaries of public responsibility in relation to water provision during the nineteenth century and into the early years of the twentieth. Nevertheless, a local government survey conducted at about the time of the First World War still found 2,160 water undertakings, well less than half of which – 786 – were municipally owned.[12] Even in 1963, nearly twenty years after the 1945 Water Act of the nationalizing Attlee government, twenty-nine private companies still provided approximately a quarter of the water supply in England and Wales. It was not until the Water Act of 1973 that the ten multi-purpose water authorities which were later to be privatized came into being. With some further relatively minor amendments in the 1983 Water Act, the stage was set for privatization.

The water industry in Wales and England was privatized in 1989, while remaining in public hands in both Scotland and Northern Ireland. The policy shared the basic unpopularity which surrounded the privatization of all public utilities but differed from electricity and telecommunications – and to a lesser extent, gas – in remaining unpopular thereafter.[13] On a monopoly basis, and with very little commercial risk, approximately 20 million domestic consumers are now supplied by the privatized companies thus created. In the absence of competition, the Conservative government looked to regulation to fill the gap. In doing so, Maloney and Richardson[14] suggest, a shift had taken place from 'the private management of public business to the public management of private business'. Ofwat, the Office of Water Industry Regulation, was thus created with a primary duty to ensure the profitability of the water companies and a secondary duty to protect the interests of customers. This hierarchy of obligations contains within it the kernel of the most fundamental change which privatization can be said to have brought about in terms of water supply. In the relevant literature, this is most often referred to as a new paradigm in which 'public goods' have been 'commodified' – that is, placed on the same basis as any other goods or services which are traded in the market-place. Guy et al.[15] explain the change in this way:

> the key shift instigated by the privatisation and liberalisation of the utility markets has been the replacement of the ethic of public service – the ideal of affordable, reliable, universal access to utility services at constant tariffs for all, irrespective of income or location. Replacing this has been the goal of profitability. The overriding aim of British utility companies today is the maximisation of profits for shareholders and (increasingly global) financial investors.

The shifting boundary between public and private ownership of water is thus one which brought fundamental alterations in its wake. Did health form part of these changes? Essentially, the case advanced here revolves around the impact of private ownership upon affordability and the growing evidence, both that increasing numbers of individual customers were unable to meet their bills and that, in a core of hard cases at least, the means developed by companies to address this situation were making matters worse rather than better. Even before such direct evidence had become available, the central connections with which this chapter is concerned, these developments had been linked by the BMA[16] in its first report in this way: on the one hand, 'access to a supply of clean water is a fundamental right and a prerequisite for good public health', while on the other, investigations were necessary because of 'concern at the potential health effects of the forthcoming privatization of the water supply industry'. It is to a more detailed exploration of these issues in the years immediately after privatization – the Conservative years – that this chapter now turns.

The Conservative Years

In the years immediately after privatization, a series of concerns came rapidly to the fore which have a direct bearing upon the key relationships between water, ownership and health. The issues to be addressed here include prices, poverty, debt, disconnection and the law.

Prices

Water prices have risen far more since privatization than in any other of the privatized household utilities. Between 1989/90 and 1994/5 the average increase in household water and sewerage bills ran to 67 per cent, more than three times as fast as inflation over the same period. A House of Commons research paper published in December 1998[17] suggests that, in terms of the most recent figures: 'Since privatisation, the average combined (water and sewerage) bill for households billed on both measured and un-measured bases has approximately doubled in cash terms, increasing by 46% in real terms.'

Rising water prices hit low-income households hardest and with proportionately greater impact than on people with higher incomes. Using average Ofwat figures, the National Consumer Council[18] suggested that whereas a household on income support in 1989/90 had to spend 2.5 per cent of disposable income on water, this would have risen, by 1994/5, to 3.2 per cent. A lone parent with an eight-year-old child spent 4 per cent of disposable income on water in 1989/90 and would spend 5 per cent in 1994/5. The combined bills for water and sewerage have been estimated by Ofwat[19] as rising to take as much as 14 per cent of the income of a single pensioner on income support by 2004–5.

The capacity of poorer households to cope with these rapidly rising bills has been affected by changes in the benefit system. Following the introduction of income support in 1988, water was excluded from the formula used in uprating calculations. It was subsequently reincluded in 1992 but the shortfall during the intervening years was never made good. During those missing years water prices rose faster than any item which is included in the calculation of the index. The government's own Social Security Advisory Committee[20] summarized the resulting position in this way: 'there remains a shortfall in the income of those receiving income related benefits as no recompense was made for the period from 1988 to 1991, although water charges increased dramatically in that time.'

A second factor which has increased the vulnerability of many more of the poorest water customers is to be found in the growing variation in prices between one water company and another since privatization. Ofwat's[21] latest price review document, for example, suggests that actual household bills for water and sewerage, in 1998–9 varied between £158 and £73 in relation to the most expensive and cheapest water companies and £229 and £102 in relation to company charges for sewerage. While privately set prices vary between one part of the country and another, publicly set benefit rates remain the same for all. A report from the Policy Studies Institute[22] concluded that 'differences in the amounts which people living in different parts of the country have to pay for basic services are significant and seem to be widening'. It found the highest charge for water to be £6.33 a week and the lowest £2.06. The highest charge for electricity was estimated at £5.99 a week and the lowest £5.04. In relation to these two privately run enterprises alone, therefore, a cash difference of £5.22 each week could exist between families in similar circumstances and with identical disposable incomes provided by the state.

Poverty, water and health
Within this general picture, certain groups of people, particularly those with health needs which increase the costs of laundry, have

been especially badly treated in the benefit system changes. Until the 1988 changes, it was possible to claim a 'laundry addition' to the basic supplementary benefit rate, where high essential use of water could be established. In the final year of that scheme 550,000 claimants received the additional payment. Were such payments still available, that figure would be unlikely to have fallen. Indeed, as other commentators have suggested: 'the figure of 550,000 claimants who might now have high essential use of water is certainly an under-estimate.'[23]

Individuals requiring help because of excess laundry costs are likely to be drawn disproportionately from those who have a physical disability – that is to say, from a group in the population whose average income is already amongst the poorest. It is estimated, for example, that 76 per cent of disabled people rely upon state benefits as their main source of income. In that study, moreover, 13 per cent of disabled adults thought they faced extra laundry charges because of their disability, and 39 per cent of families with disabled children recorded additional spending on laundry and dry cleaning.

To summarize: water costs have risen rapidly since privatization. Such costs fall particularly heavily on those groups in the population whose need for water is greatest, and these groups, in turn, are also more likely to have to rely on state benefits for their maintenance. State benefits, however, have proceeded in exactly the opposite fashion to water costs. Inadequate at the outset, benefit levels have failed to keep pace with water prices and now cover less than half the weekly cost of supply.

Debt and disconnection

From the outset water debt and disconnection have been a constant source of concern to the privatized companies. The scale of the problem is well illustrated by Herbert and Kempson[24] who report: 'during 1994 almost two million households in Britain defaulted on their water bills – nine per cent of all households in the country according to our household survey. And at the end of the year more than a million (five per cent) were currently behind with their payments.' According to Middleton and Saunders,[25]

more than a million households were behind with their water payments at the end of 1994: a year when nearly two million households defaulted on their bills. Between 1993 and 1994, more than three million pre-summons notices were issued by the water companies in England and Wales. These figures represented an increase of 900 per cent between 1990 and 1995.

In 1997, also, Graham[26] reported a recent survey in which it was found that '75% of people on Income Support . . . now have difficulty paying water bills, and that problems of water debt are rising faster than any other form of debt'. Globally, government figures suggest[27] that bad debts within the industry are currently running at about £90 million a year, or 1.5 per cent of turnover.

In the years immediately after privatization, companies attempted to respond to problems of non-payment through a vigorous application of their powers to disconnect those in debt from their domestic supply. The figures rose sharply. In the Dŵr Cymru case, for example, the number increased from 1,243 in 1989/90 to 2,938 in 1991/2. By 1992/3 the company had the second highest proportion of disconnection per 10,000 households billed of all the major companies, with a rate of 21.46 against a national average of 9.51.[28] Unsurprisingly, the juxtaposition of poor people having to go without water, and an industry making ever-growing profits proved a public relations disaster. According to the House of Commons,[29] for example, Dŵr Cymru's highest-paid director's pay has risen by 96 per cent in real terms since privatization while the company's pre-tax profits have risen by 510 per cent in cash terms, or 351 per cent in real terms, over the same period. Under pressure from the public and the regulator, the companies looked elsewhere for means of ensuring that supplies were made available only to those who were able to pay their bills.

In the space available here, only one development of the Conservative period can be discussed in any detail – the introduction of prepayment methods of purchasing water. Such devices were by no means the only – or even, arguably, the main – way in which water companies attempted to obtain payment for their services from poor people during this period. The Department of Social Security (DSS) Direct Payment scheme, for example, saw deductions from benefit for water bills rise from 67,000 in 1991 to 235,000 in 1995. Estimates suggest that up to 40 per cent of claimants on direct payment have insufficient left to meet basic daily necessities. Prepayment meters – or Budget Payment Units (BPUs) – are focused upon here because they represent an initiative which proceeded entirely from within the privatized industry itself. The units provided a means which allowed a customer to purchase a supply of water for a certain period of time – typically a week – rather than a volume of supply. Householders were provided with a 'smart' card or key which had to be taken to a charging point where it could be encoded with the credit which activated the unit located at the individual's home. Failure to purchase sufficient credit resulted in water being cut off. In the event of such 'self-disconnection' – as it became known in the industry – consumers remained liable to pay for the period of time during which they were unable to receive a supply of water. To reactivate a water prepayment device, following a period of self-disconnection, therefore, became a potentially costly and difficult business.

In Wales the Customer Services Committee (CSC) 'welcomed the initiative' of Dŵr Cymru in taking the lead in the nation-wide use of prepayment devices.[30] The company's embrace of prepayment methods was enthusiastic. In April 1994, 328 customers were paying for water in this way. At 31 January 1995, 1,136 units had been installed, a 346 per cent increase over ten months. By July 1995 the number had risen further to 2,400. At this stage its use significantly outstripped that of any other privatized company. Thus not only do prices vary between companies – with the impact which this produces upon poorer customers – but there is also, as Middleton and Saunders[31] discovered, 'significant variation between companies, in disconnection and water debt'. In terms of the public/private interface with which this chapter is concerned, it is clear that, following privatization, the policies pursued for debt recovery have varied from place to place, in a way which was not as characteristic of a publicly provided service. In the case of Dŵr Cymru, within a further eighteen months 17,800 units were in operation, more than the rest of the country put together, and the company reported that it expected that 20,000 customers would have moved to this method of payment by 31 March 1997, overtaking direct payment from benefit as the most likely payment method for those in significant debt. Despite this, the 1996/7 report from the chairman of the Wales CSC[32] contained no single observation about prepayment meters in any of their aspects.

As far as the companies are concerned, prepayment meters offered a number of key advantages. As Ernst[33] suggests:

as well as giving customers in default the facility to remain on supply, pre-payment meters (ppms) have clear advantages for the utility companies. They provide a continuous revenue stream in advance of the consumption of energy, which contrasts with the way that revenue is raised from the bulk of consumers, and they give the utilities a secured way of retrieving debt with minimal costs.

As such, these systems allow companies to escape the opprobrium which disconnection brings while circumventing other existing legal means of dealing with debt recovery and allowing water companies to leapfrog over other creditors.

For customers, however, the impact of prepayment methods was more complex. Companies relied, for the most part, on survey evidence which they had commissioned, which suggested that such devices were 'popular' amongst users and provided only on the basis of customer 'choice' – itself a more complex question than companies usually implied.[34] Other surveys, however, suggested that such satisfaction came at a high price. A MORI study, between March 1993 and July 1994, indicated that 80 per cent of households with a prepayment device had needed to use the emergency credit facility, and 10 per cent had their water supply 'shut off' completely for more than twenty-four hours because they had not recharged their water keys.[35] Notifications to local environmental health officers in the same area suggested that 273 of the 1,027 households with prepayment devices had gone without water for twenty-four hours or more. A trial of prepayment water devices carried out by Severn Trent Water in 1996 showed that 49 per cent of customers in the trial had been without a water supply after running out of emergency credit. Of those cut-offs longer than seven hours, 28 per cent 'borrowed' water, which is illegal under the Water Act; 18 per cent stored water with the attendant public health risks; and 13 per cent went without water altogether.[36] The national average for statutory disconnections at the time, as published by Ofwat, was 6.3 per 10,000 households. Birmingham City Council have calculated that should Severn Trent recommence installations to reach their original target of 10,000 households, the disconnection rate through self-disconnection would have soared to 2,140 per 10,000. The journal *Utility Week* reported in September 1996[37] that two-thirds of households using water prepayment meters experienced 'self-disconnection' during the first year in use.

Taken together, the accumulating evidence suggested that the poorest families were going without water in a way which no longer brought such information to public attention; the problem, as well as the industry, had been 'privatized'.[38] The health consequences of self-disconnection include all those which had previously been identified in relation to disconnection by the companies themselves, together with a number of others, two of which can be identified here. The first refers to the effects of volumetric metering, as a method of paying for water, which will be discussed in more detail later in this chapter. In terms of access to supply, research commissioned by Ofwat and the Department of Environment[39] suggested that metered supplies resulted in high proportions of large households and people on low incomes – and 62 per cent of those with medical conditions – believing that they needed more water than they could afford. The practical consequences were that, 'amongst social security claimants with meters 79% had cut down on baths and showers and 60% on toilet flushing. 56% did less clothes washing and 53% less washing up.' Research by the author of this chapter suggested that prepayment meters produced a similar 'shadow' effect upon their users. While cutting down on use of water provided an entirely useless way of extending the time purchased through a BPU, users nevertheless, drawing on their more general appreciation of 'meters', acted as though saving on usage would make their money go further. All the techniques reported for cutting down on water by volumetric meter users were also reported by prepayment users.

Secondly, in terms of health questions, it is important to note that self-disconnection does not carry with it the legal safeguards of notification to local authorities which has to follow disconnection directly by water companies. In research conducted by the author it became clear that the stigma associated with being without water was of a different order from being without a supply of other basic utilities, such as gas or electricity. Households which became 'self-disconnected' were themselves acutely aware of the hostility which they might attract as a result of causing potential risk to others, making the pressures to conceal difficulties all the greater. Other studies have pointed in the same direction, such as that of Middleton et al.[40] whose study of disconnected households found 'unreported health problems and suggested that people in disconnected households were less likely to be identified by health systems'. Hidden disconnection arguably presents the greatest risk of all to public health, and that risk was increased by the actions of the privatized companies.

Such was the disquiet at the spread of prepayment meters in the water industry that in February 1998 a case for judicial review was taken to the High Court by a consortium of local authorities.[41] The action was taken against the industry regulator, on the grounds that he had failed to prevent the companies from breaching their legal obligation to supply. The Judge, Mr Justice Harrison, found for the local authorities on all counts, declaring the prepayment meters illegal. The aftermath, including Dŵr Cymru's reluctant compliance with the court's judgement and the industry's attempt to circumvent the ruling through 'trickle-flow' and '2-in-1' meters are dealt with in a later section. The conclusion which this chapter reaches at the end of the Conservative years in government is as follows: the privatization settlement in the water industry had reached a point where the institutional system of checks and balances which was claimed to have been put in place at the point of privatization had almost completely failed. The companies, the regulator, the customer services committees and – if less openly – the government were all supporters of prepayment methods of making sure that no customer would be able to obtain a supply of water for which she or he would be unable to meet the bill. Coopey and Roberts[42] suggest that public ownership of water was brought about by a mixture of public health and political considerations. In the privatization of the water industry in England and Wales only one factor was of real significance. The Schumpeterian belief in the intrinsic merits of private ownership was sufficiently intense to relegate all other considerations – affordability, health and customer protection – to little more than side-issues.

New Labour

This chapter now turns to the actions and policy developments of the New Labour government of May 1997, as emerging gradually over its first two years in office. The basis of Labour's approach was summarized in the report of the party's Policy Commission on the Environment,[43] *In Trust for Tomorrow*, which declared: 'We will ensure that the actions of water companies are under public control.' This simple statement embodied an essential distinction between *public ownership* and *public control*. The Conservative Party had been actively opposed to both. The Labour Party, by the time of the 1997 election, had abandoned its long-standing commitment to the first, in preference to the second. Within that general policy framework, a number of individual measures are now clearly in place, as the remainder of this chapter will demonstrate.

Regulation and consumer representation
Labour launched an early review of regulation and consumer representation in all the privatized utilities. The results were widely regarded as disappointing. The government made no proposals to reverse the privatization policies of its predecessor. It decided to leave intact the basis of industry regulation, emphasizing the neo-liberal argument that regulation provided only a surrogate for the benefits which competition would bring in an unregulated market. The most substantial change was to place a primary duty upon the regulator to protect the interests of customers. No specific duty was included, however, to protect the interests of low-income customers. The regulators' response was to claim that, in practice, these issues had always commanded equal prominence. Consumer representation in the water industry was to be placed on a statutory basis. In the view of low-income consumer groups the change was more cosmetic than real, failing to tackle the basic failures of a system which had been demonstrably ineffective hitherto, particularly in the representation of the interests of poorer consumers.[44] The regulator, in his most recent annual report, commended the government for its recognition of 'the value of close working between the regulator and consumer bodies'.[45] Those who advocated a different arrangement, usually emphasizing the benefits of using existing public-sector organizations such as council trading standards departments, regarded the closeness of regulator and consumer representation precisely as evidence of the unsatisfactory nature of such arrangements. Labour's proposals contained no concessions to the demand of water-poverty lobbying groups that committees should be partisan in favour of low-income groups, including the representation of low-income consumers on committees.

Water prices
The New Labour government came to office with a particular proposal to fund a major public programme – the New Deal – through a windfall tax on privatized utility profits. The formula employed was claimed, by the company, to be particularly punitive in the case of Dŵr Cymru. The government also made it clear, in a general sense, that it believed that regulation had failed to strike an adequate balance between consumer and company interests. In the case of water, the results of the last price review had resulted in a 4.5 per cent real-terms increase in average household water bills and a 10.5 per cent real-terms increase in average sewerage charges.[46] With considerable fanfare, the regulator announced, in July 1999, that the settlement for the coming four years would produce an average 14 per cent decrease in water prices during the first twelve months, even though they were set to rise again in real terms towards the end of the five-year price review period.[47]

Two important caveats have to be entered against these much-vaunted claims. Firstly, the figures provided refer only to *average* household bills, with very little evidence available in order to assess the impact upon particular groups in the population. Secondly, the review appears to have abandoned entirely any attempt to equalize the level of charges between one part of the country and another. As established earlier in this chapter, price differentials are the product of the shifting private/public boundary in water provision. The cost-reflective policies pursued by companies since privatization, with the enthusiastic support of the regulator, have produced the widening gaps which consumers, according to the accident of geography, face between one part of the country and another. The policies pursued by New Labour show no sign of equalizing this poverty lottery by public action.

Prepayment meters
New Labour's record on prepayment metering and other similar devices is amongst the strongest elements in this policy field. The decision to make such devices unlawful had to be pursued against the opposition of the industry, the regulator and the CSCs. The Welsh CSC, for example, had reaffirmed its support for the use of Budget Payment Units at its meeting of 13 March 1997.[48] In his 1997 Annual Report Mr Byatt remained grudgingly opposed to the disappearance of prepayment, recording the High Court case

which found Ofwat to have been acting illegally in this way: 'Despite safeguards and evidence that customers found BPUs to be a convenient method of payment, six local authorities objected to their use and sought Judicial Review in the High Court of the Director's decision not to prevent water companies offering this payment option.'[49]

With the passage of the Water Act, which received the royal assent on 30 June 1999, not only were prepayment meters brought to an end, but disconnection of domestic water supplies for non-payment of bills was also made illegal in Wales and England, bringing them back into line with the situation which had always appertained in Scotland and Northern Ireland. Needless to say, the move had again been opposed by the trinity of companies, regulator and customer committees, with Ian Byatt plainly lining up with those who believed that 'without the threat of disconnection, reluctant payers would not meet their bills'.[50] As a result, Ofwat's annual publication of company disconnection figures came to an end in June 1999, when it reported that nine companies had already anticipated the new requirements by not disconnecting any households in the year April 1998 to March 1999, with a further twelve reporting lower numbers of disconnections than in the previous year. Dŵr Cymru, by contrast, recorded the second-largest rise in the number of domestic disconnections over the same period amongst all the privatized companies and a pattern of rising figures over a three-year period.[51] Commenting on the passage of the Act into law, the minister responsible for the water industry in England, Michael Meacher commented in terms which lie at the heart of the argument which this chapter presents:

> Maintaining an uninterrupted supply of water is a benchmark of civilisation, on which life and good health depend . . . It is totally unacceptable that anyone should be deprived of a water supply in their home simply because of an inability to pay.[52]

The changes in relation to disconnection thus emerge as a significant change in the operating environment of such an essential service as supply of water. Before leaving the issue altogether, however, it is worth recalling the warning of Martin Fitch that the concentration upon disconnection itself distorts essential debates in this area, focusing upon the 'way we process the poor', rather than upon ways in which poverty itself might be addressed.[53] If the only effect of the Water Act changes is to be a new twist in the race to develop technological devices which force water bills to the top of poor people's spending priorities, or to turn the companies' attentions to more oppressive ways of pursuing bills short of disconnection – county court proceedings, bailiffs and so on – then the gains of the Act may yet prove illusory.

Trickle-flow

When it became clear that prepayment methods were to be unavailable to the industry, some companies, and Dŵr Cymru[54] in particular, set off instead in the direction of what came to be known as 'trickle-flow' meters. The system, as the name implies, involves the installation of valves which allows a much-reduced flow of water to those customers who had failed to pay their bills. Six months after the High Court judgement in relation to prepayment meters, Dŵr Cymru had installed some 1,000 trickle-flow meters in Wales, as part of a plan to move rapidly to 3,000.[55]

When such devices had been considered by North West Water, Liverpool City Council's Environmental Health Service took the view that 'trickle-flow' potentially represented a more serious hazard than a straight disconnection. The service was particularly concerned about the likely dangers to certain types of heating systems, particularly older systems which were not regularly maintained (this includes 'multi-point' systems as well as central heating). Such problems are commonplace in houses in multiple occupation – exactly the type of property where prepayment meters were most likely to be installed. British Gas took the same view as Environmental Health, leading to North West Water discounting 'trickle-flow' as a viable option.

When technicians in Liverpool City Council's Architect's Department carried out a series of experiments on the practical implementation of trickle-flow using technical information supplied by North West Water, they found that the flow rates proposed meant that it would not be possible to run a shower, a washing machine or a combination boiler central heating system (effectively disconnecting the consumer's main heating source). A toilet cistern would take twenty minutes to fill and the amount of water supplied would just about be sufficient to boil a kettle or wash one's hands and face.

Despite this evidence, and the views of the regulator that trickle-flow meters were covered by the same set of arguments which the High Court had developed in outlawing prepayment meters, Dŵr Cymru insisted on going ahead with their installation. It was not until the government made it clear that such devices would also be legislated against in the Water Bill that the company altered its policy. Government intentions in this regard were set out in the *Response to Consultation* document provided by the Department of the Environment, Transport and the Regions (DETR), declaring that it does not 'believe that they provide sufficient assurances against the concerns over public health which are at the heart of the Government's water charging policy'.

As Fitch[56] would have predicted, however, the actions of the companies were not at an end. In Wales, Hyder, the parent company of Dŵr Cymru, had in 1996 acquired ownership of the privatized electricity supply company, SWALEC. A number of concerns had already been expressed about the powerful position which multi-utility companies would occupy in the lives of their customers, including anxiety that information about debt to one arm of the parent company might be shared with another. Now Dŵr Cymru proposed a means of organizing payment of their water charges through the far more extensive network of electricity prepayment meters (ppms) inherited through SWALEC. Within the industry, the approach became known as the 2-in-1 system and involved automatically depriving people of their electricity as well if they failed to keep up payments for water. Negotiations about the new system began between SWALEC and the electricity regulator, Offer, early in 1998. Offer became concerned that the use of electricity ppms for this purpose could result – in the event that customers did not recharge their meters – in their supply of electricity being disconnected because of water debt. By mid-June the director general had concluded that it was not reasonable for electricity supply to be cut off by self-disconnection in the circumstances in question. SWALEC was told by the regulator that it should therefore take all reasonable steps to discontinue the scheme as soon as possible. This was reiterated in August 1998, but with little apparent effect. By the time the matter came to the attention of the secretary of state at the Department of Trade and Industry in October 1998, as many as 3,000 customers were said to be paying for water in this way. In the following month, SWALEC informed Offer that, in its view, the concerns which had been expressed were misplaced. It proposed issuing proceedings for a judicial declaration to resolve the question. In the meantime, it gave assurances that, pending the outcome of declaration proceedings, no new customers would be taken onto the scheme. It was left to the courts, once again, to declare the system illegal.[57]

In terms of the central issue of public and private responsibilities which runs through this volume, the history of prepayment, trickle-flow and 2-in-1 meters casts an instructive light upon the reliance of government upon the powers of the regulator in dealing with private companies. In the first two cases, the regulator quite directly took the side of the companies against those individuals and organizations who had questioned the legality and morality of providing water in this way. In all three cases, the companies' response to regulatory requirements raises questions about the effectiveness of regulators' powers. Dŵr Cymru seems to have ignored for several months the water regulators' instructions to take out or disarm BPUs. The company equally acted in open defiance of the advice which the regulator provided in relation to trickle-flow. SWALEC delayed acting on the regulator's advice to stop the 2-in-1 scheme. The balance of power in the new settlement between private and public in the provision of utility services seems unambiguously weighted in favour of the former.

Volumetric metering
If the Water Act of the New Labour government provided a number of real gains in terms of access to water for the most vulnerable households, the same measure provided at least one substantial blow to those who had campaigned against the effects of privatization on poorest consumers. In opposition, Labour had declared: 'We will outlaw water disconnections for residential properties and ban compulsory water metering.'[58] Now, in contradiction of that stance, the Act provided a new impetus to the installation of volumetric meters for water, a process which, as table 10.1 illustrates, had already been under way for some time.

The detail of the different ways in which volumetric meters could now be demanded by those who wished them, and imposed upon others whether they wanted them or not, need not detain us here. There is little dispute that the Act will add impetus to the 'creeping meterization' which has come to be characteristic of the

Table 10.1 Metered households as percentage of households receiving water supplies

1990/1	1992/3	1994/5	1996/7	1998/9
2%	4%	7%	11%	14%

Source: House of Commons Research Report (1998), 14.

industry since privatization.[59] The health consequences of such a development, however, do require attention, and fall into two main categories. Firstly, the effects of volumetric metering do not fall only upon those who purchase a supply of water in this way. The total income extracted by the companies from consumers has to remain the same, whatever methods of payment happen to be shared between them. The effect of this has already been seen in the different fates of measured-supply users who have seen their bills actually fall in real terms (1998/9 prices) by 2 per cent since privatization, while unmeasured bills have increased by 48 per cent.[60]

Thus, as those consumers who stand to benefit financially – single people in expensive properties, for example – switch to volumetric meters, the money which they save has to be made up by increasing the bills of those who remain on an unmeasured supply. As the latter are more likely to be poorer households, living in the least expensive properties, the effect is regressive, shifting costs from those who can afford them the most to those who can afford them the least.

Secondly, the effects of being obliged to purchase water by volume have already been demonstrated to act to the detriment of vulnerable households, especially in the case of large families or those whose particular health needs led to heavy demands for water. A discussion paper published by the Rowntree Foundation in June 1997 concluded: 'metered tariffs discriminate against low-income households who need above average amounts of domestic water, including those with young children or older people with incontinence problems or other disabilities requiring intensive water-use.'[61] A study for the Save the Children Fund,[62] for example, found that those with meters paid 4 per cent of their income on water charges, compared with a UK average figure of 1 per cent.

The study was carried out on two newly built estates, new buildings being one of the instances where volumetric metering is compulsorily installed. Fifty families, or 70 per cent of the sample, 'were taking measures to reduce their use of water'.[63] Noting that the right of access to water is specified in the 1989 United Nations Convention on the Rights of the Child, ratified by the UK government in 1991, the report showed that larger families paid proportionately higher charges and that the impact upon children included fewer baths/showers and less washing of clothes and less flushing of the toilet. The fund suggested that 'the long term health risks associated with such rationing of water included increased risk of dysentery, hepatitis A and body lice', while the increased parental anxieties which were associated with struggling to pay for water also produced a direct impact upon children in the family.

The 1999 Water Act recognizes some of the difficulties which would be faced by such families in properties where volumetric metering has become compulsory. The Act proposes offering low-income customers in these circumstances the option of charge by average use. Unfortunately, despite the passage of the Act into law, the government has, at the time of writing, yet to publish even a consultation paper on the practical implementation of this proposal. In the meantime, while a series of potential problems have already been identified by consumer groups, the principle upon which the concession has been made – that 'people with designated medical conditions' require protection – further confirms the key contention of a relationship between water, health and mode of display upon which this paper is based.

Protecting vulnerable groups
One of the most direct ways in which the New Labour government has revived the connection between water and health, and emphasized the importance of the public/private boundary, is to be found in the specific protections which the Water Act proposes for vulnerable groups who find themselves compulsorily supplied with a volumetric meter. Under clause 5 of the Act the secretary of state is empowered to make regulations to define the groups to be offered protection and the precise nature of the support they should receive. The minister responsible, Michael Meacher, set out the government's thinking, in the House of Commons on 7 December 1998 (Hansard col. 45):

We propose that protection should be available to families with three or more children in receipt of one of the following benefits: income support; income-based JSA, family credit; disability working allowance, housing and council-tax benefit.

For the second group, we propose that protection should be offered to those with conditions such as desquamating or weeping skin diseases, incontinence, abdominal stomas, ileostomies and colostomies, and renal failure requiring home dialysis. We propose that to gain protection, customers would have to certify to the water companies that they suffer from one of these conditions that causes them to need an unusually high amount of water.

While the connection between water and health was thus firmly established, the government was also anxious not to place any burden upon the private companies through the protection it sought for vulnerable individuals. In its *Response to Consultation* paper, for example, it made it clear that, 'the Government does not intend to place unnecessary burdens on water companies in offering protection to customers with special needs'.[64] The tension between public welfare and private provision of essential services was once again apparent and remained so in both the Utilities Act of 2000 (which contained a provision empowering the secretary of state to require companies to adjust tariffs in favour of low-income consumers, accompanied by assurances that it was most unlikely ever to be invoked)[65] and the 'water benefit', introduced in April 2001.

What verdict might be offered on the emerging New Labour policy approach to water issues? Fitch[66] perhaps sums it up best as caught in the 'ambiguity of a softening of budget discipline (ending disconnection) together with a determination to press ahead with marketisation . . . Water companies remain profit driven and will be anxious to deploy alternative sanctions for debt recovery.'

Two further items remain for brief consideration in this account of water, health and ownership issues at the end of the twentieth century. These issues straddle the years since privatization and both provide a relatively specialist insight into the general questions explored here.

Fire risk
As is the case in relation to so many risks in contemporary Britain, the distribution of difficulty experienced by citizens does not fall

equally across all groups. As Chandler et al.[67] suggest, 'if you are an unemployed city dweller living in overcrowded, shared accommodation, you are much more likely to find yourself the victim of a domestic fire, than the average UK householder.' Two issues arise in relation to privatization, water and health in this regard. Firstly, families with lower incomes tend to use less safe forms of heating (open fires and portable heaters) and, as they are more likely to have their gas or electricity supplies cut off – either directly or through being unable to afford to feed prepayment meters – they therefore resort to using more dangerous alternatives, such as candles for lighting. Evidence exists of an increased incidence of household fires caused in this way, and of firefighters experiencing additional difficulties in providing emergency services because of tampering with water supplies by those cut off from domestic supplies in some disadvantaged areas.

The second instance arises from the pressure put upon water companies by the New Labour government, to address the problem of loss of water through leakages. Some months after the Downing Street Water Summit in May 1997, it emerged that some companies had acted to tackle leakage by reducing water pressure in the supply networks. Fire chiefs in Leicestershire, for example, reported having to obtain water from a canal because of insufficient pressure in a hydrant.[68] While companies denied that they were 'cutting leaks on the cheap', emergency talks were convened between the Home Office, the Department of the Environment, the Local Government Association and the water companies, in order to obtain the 'absolute assurances' which government ministers demanded that the leakage problem was not being tackled in this way.

Fluoridation
The whole of the fluoridation debate is far too wide and detailed to be summarized in the space available in this chapter. One aspect, however, is of particular interest: the extent to which changing ownership of the industry has made a difference to adding fluoride to water supplies. The health claims for fluoridation are that it provides the single most effective way of improving the dental health of the nation, particularly children. According to the Acheson Report,[69] a sixfold difference exists in dental health between the best and worst parts of the United Kingdom, a pattern

which closely reflects the pattern of poverty and affluence across the country. Acheson also suggests that the health gap is widening while, unlike almost all other diseases, the government has a simple, cheap and effective measure at its disposal which could make a radical difference. Currently some 10 per cent of the population has fluoride added to water, above the natural levels, almost all of which was introduced during the 1970s by local authorities which then controlled the water supply. Not a single privatized water company has been willing to introduce fluoridation since transfer of ownership, despite requests from more than sixty health authorities. Companies have been unwilling to face the potential claims for damages which might be laid at their door if fluoridation were to prove problematic. In December 1998 Northumbrian Water successfully resisted, through the lawcourts, a local authority attempt to force the introduction of fluoridation throughout the northern region.

Whatever the questions of civil liberty which the issue engenders, the health claims for fluoridation are serious ones. The different patterns of its application, however, are not best explained by either libertarian or physical considerations. It is the switch from public to private ownership which defines the changed outcome and with it, as many would argue, the private interests of their shareholders above the health gains of the public at large.

Postscript: Is there a 'Welsh Way' for Water?

This chapter has concentrated upon a disputatious period in the delivery of water services in Wales. The events considered, however, did not exhaust the capacity for controversy contained in the industry. Labour's tightening of the regulatory regime produced an impact on water companies throughout England and Wales, but appeared to make a particular impression upon the Welsh Water company, Dŵr Cymru, and its parent company, Hyder, which entered into a period of falling profits, declining stockmarket confidence and growing corporate uncertainty. The company appeared to have achieved the impossible, in turning the monopoly supply of a basic necessity into a risky business.

From late 1999 to August 2000 an unseemly battle was waged for new ownership of the company, now with the additional

'complication' (as some commentators put it) of the presence of
the National Assembly for Wales, 'anxiously scrutinising the
horizon for signs of approaching invaders'.[70] On 11 August 2000,
the London stockmarket take-over panel invoked, for the first time,
a procedure intended to introduce an element of finality and
seemliness into a bidding system which appeared to be dangerously
out of control and open-ended. The American-owned company
Western Power Distribution (WPD) emerged victorious. Its problems were not over, however. In October 2000 the courts ruled that
its contracting plans breached British and UK regulations and
would have to be reopened to tender. In November 2000 a new
solution emerged through Glas Cymru, an organization which
advertised itself as a Welsh-based, not-for-profit company, limited
by guarantee, in which members would take on the corporate
governance role of shareholders. It intended, from the outset, to set
a self-imposed impediment, contained in its covenants, preventing
the company from diversifying out of water. It claimed that, by
raising the money needed to finance the industry's statutory
investment programme through debt, rather than equity, it would
be able both to reduce costs and the bills charged to customers.

A second joint meeting of the National Assembly's Economic
Development and Environment, Transport and Planning Committees was held on 15 November 2000. Speaking on behalf of the
company, Geraint Talfan Davies opened by reminding members:
'We all know that the water issue resonates in Wales in a way that it
does not do anywhere else in the UK.' It was, said another
contributor, both 'a highly emotive subject and a valuable
economic resource'. The company's plans were

> based on the premise of exposing the fact that the water industry is a
> low risk business. It provides an essential public service. It is a
> monopoly . . . The company will have a local focus on priorities in
> Wales and, because it does not have equity shareholders, it is our belief
> that it will be more open and accountable than is currently the case
> with some of the equity-owned companies. We have no reason for
> secrecy and I think that that is a major benefit for this company.

Despite the fact that Glas Cymru's bid was headed by former
Treasury permanent secretary, Lord Burns, the initiative was
opposed by what the *Guardian*[71] described as an 'unlikely alliance'

of central government departments. The Treasury had already successfully opposed plans to turn Scotland's municipally owned water companies into mutuals. It now combined with the Department of Trade and Industry and the DETR to resist the Glas Cymru proposals, largely on the basis that the absence of shareholders would militate against incentives and efficiency. Regulators, too, proved sceptical. *The Financial Times* on 23 January 2001[72] reported that the electricity industry regulator, Callum McCarthy, had opposed the use of debt rather than equity on the grounds that such a structure lacked the incentives necessary to improve efficiency.

On the other side of the political equation, the deal secured the active support of many National Assembly for Wales politicians and the background encouragement of the first minister, Rhodri Morgan, who emphasized the importance of the proposal being given a fair hearing. A meeting with the Ofwat regulator, Philip Fletcher, produced an understanding, set out in the regulator's position paper on the proposed acquisition of Dŵr Cymru by Glas Cymru,[73] that their consultation had shown 'broad support in Wales for Glas, notably from the National Assembly for Wales'. Against this background, Glas Cymru acquired Welsh Water on 11 May 2001 in a deal which involved paying WPD £1 for Dŵr Cymru, while assuming £1.85 billion in net debt from the parent company, Hyder. A bridging loan was acquired to buy back the Hyder debt, before a bond issue raised the capital necessary to refinance the deal. While sharing some of the conventional disquiet at the capacity of the company to raise sufficient low-interest bond market funding, and at the absence of efficiency incentives in the proposed company structure, Ofwat nevertheless gave the go-ahead to the acquisition, subject to a number of caveats, particularly those in relation to incentivization. In a final letter of 11 July, the director general gave his approval in these terms: 'In the absence of shareholder pressure, it is intended that the approach you have taken to rebates and the structure of executive directors' remuneration should provide incentives to achieve continuing greater efficiency.'[74]

Despite the qualms of traditional financial interests, the bond issue was 70 per cent oversubscribed. Two billion pounds was raised on the British and continental bond markets, drawing seventy-nine investors. One billion pounds of this sum was triple-A rated, a market assessment which placed the company in the very lowest risk category, and thus able to borrow money at the lowest rates of interest. By contrast, Dŵr Cymru in its final and most troubled stages had been rated as triple-B minus, the lowest level of investment grade rating. The practical effect was to cut the annual cost of capital to just over 4 per cent, rather than the normal 6 per cent. This, by itself, saved the company £50 million annually, more than its entire salary bill.

As to incentives, the three executive members on the nine-strong board are able to double their £125,000 salaries through bonuses 'tied to customer service performance, water quality, reduced gearing, credit rating and other criteria'.[75] Will Hutton[76] suggested that the successful launch of the Glas Cymru model had provided a 'third way' in utility organization, replacing both public ownership and privatization models with a new 'public interest' form of ownership. An essential part of Glas Cymru's successful seeking after a high investment grade was an outsourcing strategy for operations and maintenance functions on the one hand and customer services on the other. By transferring financial operating risks to outsourced providers, the risks to Glas Cymru were reduced and the prospects of being able to borrow money through low-cost bonds was enhanced. The practical consequences of this decision were to retain a core workforce at Glas Cymru itself of some 120 people, while 1,800 people were to be subject to the outsourcing contracts. The potential impact upon this larger number were soon apparent. By 11 June, the then economic development minister, Michael German, was in talks with directors of Glas Cymru to find out more about some 185 job losses announced in the previous week by United Utilities, winners of the outsourcing contract for operations and maintenance. The company advised that the job losses were a consequence of the Ofwat targets to reduce operating costs by 5 per cent per year for the next five years, and were not a result of the acquisition. However, it was also made clear that that long-term employment in the business, including the outsourced activities, would depend on the efficient level of costs for the water business – in other words, that further job losses might yet follow.

At the time of writing, Glas Cymru's actual performance remains at a very early stage. Yet, in reporting its first half-yearly results in November 2001 the company recorded an underlying surplus for the period of £11.8 million, all of which, in the nature of a not-for-profit arrangement, was retained in the business. Pre-tax profit for the six months was 3 per cent higher than forecast. Reductions in household bills were confirmed, while the target for establishing a contingency reserve against unexpected future difficulties was already expected to be exceeded.[77] In December 2001 the company received the award for the most innovative deal of the year by the *International Financial Review*. The award citation suggested that the deal 'was a ground breaker in all kinds of ways . . . The deal's structure looks set to provide a financing solution for a range of utilities and for water companies in particular.'[78]

Conclusion

The issues considered in this chapter do not lead to a neat set of interlocking or causal relationships. Some themes, however, do emerge. The connection between water and the public interest which came under concerted attack from the high reaches of government during the late 1980s and 1990s has been replaced by an understanding both of the risk which individuals face when going without a sufficient supply of clean water and of the risk which such individuals pose to public and community health more generally. Such a recognition is explicitly identified by the New Labour administration as the rationale which underpins a number of its main Water Act reforms.[79]

The impact of water privatization questions upon health is less settled. It will be apparent to readers of this volume that, while the privatization policies of the Thatcher government are often identified as landmark events, they also have to be understood as part of far deeper and more long-standing patterns of changing responsibilities between public and private spheres.[80] It is the contention of this chapter that there are inevitable consequences which lie outside their own boundaries when private firms pursue the profits which are their basic *raison d'être*. O'Donnell and Sawyer[81] suggest that the essential contrast between the public and private modes of operation can be summarized as 'Public owner-ship will have wider objectives than private ownership: ultimately the former is concerned with the promotion of the general social

interest and the latter with profits.' In this sense, the questions of
fire hazard, fluoridation, debt and disconnection are altered by the
modified boundary of public/private ownership in the water
industry in Wales and its generation of an outcome in which it was
clearly to the profit-enhancing advantage of the supplier to squeeze
the cost consequences of their policy decisions into the public
sphere.

While commercial rather than social pressures led to the demise
of Dŵr Cymru, it remains instructive that the public debate in
Wales concerning its replacement revolved around the core
question of how far it is possible to deliver publicly desirable goals
such as social inclusion, community safety and well-being through
a market system based upon profit-driven companies. To suggest
that the jury remains out on the prospects of a 'public-interest'
solution, such as that advanced by Glas Cymru, is not a form of
academic equivocation, but rather a genuine reflection of the
fluctuations in the contemporary state of policy-making in this
essential field.

Notes

[1] Customer Service Committee for Wales (1994), *Annual Report, 1993–94*
(Cardiff, Ofwat).

[2] This volume, ch. 2.

[3] Department of Health (1999), *On the State of the Public Health: The Annual
Report of the Chief Medical Officer of the Department of Health for the Year
1997* (London, Department of Health).

[4] GAIA (1996), *Freshwater Resources* (Global Environment Information
Systems, http:/www.ess.co.at).

[5] See, for example, Waddams-Price, C. (1997), 'Regulating for fairness:
competition in the utilities can hurt the poor unless great care is taken', *New
Economy*, 4, 10.

[6] British Medical Association (1994), *Water: A Vital Resource* (London, BMA).

[7] Ibid., p. 36.

[8] Ibid.

[9] *Independent* (1996), 'Rebuff on water cuts' (20 August).

[10] Middleton, J. and Saunders, P. (1997), 'Paying for water', *Journal of Public
Health Medicine*, 19, 109.

[11] This volume, ch. 2.

[12] Ofwat (1993), *Privatisation and History of the Water Industry*, Information
Note 18 (Birmingham, Ofwat).

[13] See, for example, Taylor, B. (1991), 'Interim report: economic outlook', in
R. Jowell (ed.), *British Social Attitudes 9th Report* (Dartmouth, Social and

Community Planning Research); Heath, A. and McMahon, D. (1992), 'Changes in values', in R. Jowell (ed.), *British Social Attitudes 10th Report* (Dartmouth, Social and Community Planning Research).

[14] Maloney, W. and Richardson, J. (1995), *Managing Policy Change in Britain: The Politics of Water* (Edinburgh, Edinburgh University Press).

[15] Guy, S., Graham, S. and Marvin, S. (1997), 'Splintering networks: cities and technical networks in 1990s Britain', *Urban Studies*, 34, 203.

[16] BMA, *Water*, p. 2.

[17] House of Commons (1998), *Water Industry Bill*, Research Paper 98/117, p. 16.

[18] National Consumer Council (NCC) (1994), *Water Price Controls: Key Customer Concerns* (London, NCC).

[19] Ofwat (1993), *Paying for Quality: The Political Perspective* (Birmingham, Ofwat).

[20] Social Security Advisory Committee (1992).

[21] Ofwat (1999), *The 1999 Periodic Review: Final Determinations* (Birmingham, Ofwat).

[22] Kempson, E. and Bennett, F. (1997), *Local Living Costs* (London, Policy Studies Institute).

[23] NCC, *Water Price Controls*, p. 11.

[24] Herbert, A. and Kempson, E. (1995), *Water Debt and Disconnection* (London, Policy Studies Institute).

[25] Middleton and Saunders, 'Paying for water', 108.

[26] Graham, S. (1997), 'Liberalised utilities, new technologies and urban social polarization: the UK experience', *European Urban and Regional Studies*, 4, 135–50.

[27] DETR (1998), *Water Charging in England and Wales: A Consultation Paper* (London, HMSO).

[28] BMA, *Water*, pp. 20–1.

[29] House of Commons, *Water Industry Bill*, p. 12.

[30] CSC for Wales (1995), Minutes of twenty-second meeting, 30 March 1995 (Cardiff, Ofwat).

[31] Middleton and Saunders, 'Paying for water', 108.

[32] CSC for Wales (1997), Minutes of the thirtieth meeting, 13 March (Cardiff, Ofwat).

[33] Ernst, J. (1994), *Whose Utility? The Social Impact of Public Utility Privatization and Regulation in Britain* (Milton Keynes, Open University Press), p. 145.

[34] See Drakeford, M. (1997), 'Poverty and privatisation', *Critical Social Policy*, 17, 115–32.

[35] MORI (1994), *Electricity Services: The Customer Perspective* (London, MORI).

[36] House of Commons, *Water Industry Bill*, p. 25.

[37] *Utility Week* (1996), 'Prepayment and self-disconnection', 9 September.

[38] Drakeford, 'Poverty and privatisation'; Drakeford, M. (1998) 'Debt and disconnection in the privatized utilities', *Contemporary Wales*, 11, 149–66.

[39] Atkins Planning and Management Consultants (1992), *The Social Impact of Water Metering: A Report to the Department of the Environment and Office of Water Supplies* (London, Department of the Environment).

[40] Middleton, J., Saunders, P. and Corson, J. (1994) 'Water disconnection and disease', *Lancet*, 344, 62.

[41] For a fuller account of this episode, see Drakeford, M. (1998), 'Water regulation and pre-payment meters', *Journal of Law and Society*, 25, 588–602.

[42] This volume, ch. 2.

[43] Labour Party (1994), *In Trust for Tomorrow* (London, Labour Party).

[44] See, for example, Butterworth, T. (1995), *Off Who? Off What? Off Where? A Review of the Utility Regulator's Role in Protecting the Interests of Consumers* (Exeter, Trading Standards Department, Devon County Council).

[45] Ofwat (1998), *Director General's Annual Report 1997* (Birmingham, Ofwat).

[46] Ibid.

[47] Ofwat (1999), *1999 Periodic Review*.

[48] CSC Wales (1997), *Minutes*.

[49] Ofwat (1999), *1999 Periodic Review*.

[50] Ofwat (1998), *Director General's Annual Report*.

[51] Ofwat (1999), *1999 Periodic Review*.

[52] DETR (1998), 'Meacher launches new regime for water charging' (DETR press release, November, 975/99).

[53] Fitch, M. (1998), 'The implications for disadvantaged customers of service provision by multi-utilities' (advice note for the Local Government Anti-Poverty Forum).

[54] Dŵr Cymru (1995), *A Report on the Trial of the Fresh Start Watercard System within the Cardiff Area* (Cardiff, Welsh Water).

[55] National Local Government Forum against Poverty (NLGFAP) (1998), *Water Prepayment Devices/Trickle Flow Meters* (Cardiff, NLGFAP).

[56] Fitch (1998), 'Implications'.

[57] Fitch, M. (2001) 'Does "public utilities" mean anything any more?', *Poverty*, 108 (Winter).

[58] Labour Party (1994), *In Trust for Tomorrow*.

[59] For a more general account of the debates surrounding different methods of paying for water, see Thackray, J. E. (1997), *Paying for Household Water Services*, Social Policy Research 115 (York, Joseph Rowntree Foundation).

[60] House of Commons (1998), *Water Industry Bill*.

[61] Thackray (1997), *Paying for Household Water Services*.

[62] Cunninghame, C., Griffin, J. and Laws, S. (1994) *Water Tight: The Impact of Water Metering on Low-Income Families* (London, Save the Children).

[63] Ibid., p. 2.

[64] DETR (1998), *Water Charging in England and Wales: Response to Consultation* (London, DETR).

[65] Fitch (2001) 'Does "public utilities" mean anything?'

[66] Ibid.

[67] Chandler, Chapman and Hollington (1993) in *Fire Prevention* no. 172.

[68] *Financial Times* (1998), 'Government may act over water pressure cuts' (17 March).

[69] Acheson, D. (1998), *Independent Inquiry into Inequalities in Health Report* (London, HMSO).

[70] *Guardian* (1999), 'No hiding place for utilities' (7 December).

[71] *Guardian* (2001), 'Water deal blocked' (10 January).

[72] *Financial Times* (2001), 'Glas Cymru faces sceptical regulator' (23 January).

[73] Ofwat (2001), *Position Paper on the Proposed Acquisition of Dŵr Cymru Cyfyngedig by Glas Cymru Cygyngedig* (Birmingham, Ofwat).

[74] Ofwat (2001), 'Glas Cymru's acquisition of Dŵr Cymru: Ofwat's six conditions' (Birmingham, Ofwat).

[75] *Guardian* (2001), 'Glas Cymru sets trend by tapping bond market' (11 May).

[76] Hutton, W. (2001), 'Blair's new world vision could see our disastrous railway system back on track', *Observer*, 7 October.

[77] Glas Cymru (2001), 'Interim results for the six months to 30 September 2001' (press release, 19 November).

[78] Glas Cymru (2001), 'Glas Cymru deal named world's top deal of 2001' (Press release, 11 December).

[79] See, for example, Mullin, C. (1999), 'Fairness and affordability at heart of government's water charging policy' (Department of Environment, Transport and the Regions, 811/99).

[80] Drakeford, M. (1999), *Social Policy and Privatisation* (London, Longman).

[81] O'Donnell, K. and Sawyer, M. (1998), *A Future for Public Ownership* (London, Unison).

11

Contrasting Perspectives of Inequalities in Health and in Medical Care

DAVID GREAVES

Introduction

Condorcet (1743–94), a French philosopher of the Enlightenment, 'believed that society was made up of homogeneous individuals all born equal under the law'.[1] Such ideas fuelled the French Revolution and led to the production of a citizen's charter of health for all its people. However, as Dorothy Porter comments, 'Democratic rhetoric on health citizenship failed to translate into reality in any late Enlightenment state',[2] and this included France. No doubt there were in part sound practical reasons for this, but it was also because conceptual understandings of health and illness, which in the eighteenth century were still influenced largely by humoral ideas (involving the maintenance of a balance in the body between the four humours: blood, phlegm, black bile and yellow bile), were not consonant with the notion of equality. The Enlightenment commitment was then to political and economic equality, but did not encompass biological equality. Thus it was only gradually in the first half of the nineteenth century that equality in bodily health emerged as a new conceptual notion, as part of the emerging biomedical theory which paralleled the decline of humoralism. The central feature of biomedical theory is that it focuses on a mechanistic understanding of the body as the only true and scientific account of medical knowledge.

Perhaps for the first time in history, measurable value was being placed on the health of each and every citizen in a society. But, at the same time, how health was to be arrived at, recognised, and, more important, what it was *for*, were being construed in terms of medical intervention. This might be said to be an account of health characteristic of modern industrial societies.[3]

What this suggests is that by this time, a number of new assumptions about equality, relating to both political and medical ideas, had evolved in tandem. These were part of a wider shift in ideas relating to what is now understood as modernity (see chapter 1), and in relation to medicine and health care conveyed the following notions:

(a) that *equality in health* is both meaningful in practice and a desirable goal, so that by implication *inequalities in health* are undesirable;

(b) that *equality in medical care* (or more strictly equity) is both meaningful in practice and a desirable goal, so that by implication *inequalities in medical care* are undesirable; and

(c) that both *equality in health and in medical care* are becoming seen as public responsibilities.

Equality and Inequalities in Health and in Medical Care

During the eighteenth century and in earlier times, illness was regarded as a deviation from an individual's own natural state, so that the illness of any one person was not regarded as exactly equivalent to that of any other. By the late nineteenth century illness (and disease even more so) had come to be regarded as a deviation from a normal state, in which the condition of each person with the same medical disorder was seen to be the same, and this understanding still prevails today. Hence the idea of equality and inequality of health, illness and disease is embedded in this theoretical notion of a normal state. This shift in understanding between the eighteenth and nineteenth centuries can be seen as part of wider changes occurring in Britain, described in chapter 1, and relating to the development of what is now understood as emerging ideas of modernity, which were fuelled by the Enlightenment.

In the eighteenth century and earlier, health and illness were also conceptualized as being different for different social groups. An illustration of this can be found in recent comparisons that have been made of the heights of military recruits in Britain at age fourteen years, for which there are continuous records for the past 200 years. These show that in 1800 those who came from wealthy families and were to become officers, were on average 7–8 inches taller than those from poorer families, who were recruited to the ranks.[4] Indeed the average difference was so great that there would have been very little overlap in height between the two groups. Now the general assumption at the time was that officers were not just socially but also physically superior, and this was a natural state that it was not possible to alter. So on this understanding the idea of physical equality between those of higher and lower social standing would have been incoherent.[5] However, such notions changed radically in the nineteenth century, although they did not disappear altogether. For example, in the late nineteenth century and early twentieth century eugenics became a widely held ideology that was reliant on the assumption that the characteristics of different racial and social groups were not only culturally but biologically fixed. Earlier in the nineteenth century, though, the idea of such immutable bodily types, some of whom were naturally superior, had been largely overturned as a prerequisite to the establishment and implementation of goals relating to equality of bodily health and illness.

In the eighteenth century, there were no universally established standards of medical care, and hence there was a great variety of provision without any notion that a particular form of care was clearly superior for everyone. Porter argues that there was a pluralist medical scene, characterized by almost complete freedom to practise, which presented genuine alternatives to sufferers. Thus there was a medical market-place limited largely by the ability to pay. In this climate resorting to 'regular' practitioners, 'quacks', lay healers or self-medication was commonly regarded as being much on a level and so a matter of personal preference in each situation that arose. Even consultations with animal doctors were not uncommon.[6] However, by the late nineteenth century, all these ideas had been overturned, and this was also dependent on the gradual shift in allegiance from humoral to biomedical conceptions of health, illness and disease, which was accompanied by changes in both the profession of medicine, and society more generally.

This transformation is eloquently demonstrated by Anthony Trollope in his novel *Dr Thorne*, which was first published in 1858.[7] This was the same year in which the General Medical Council came into being in Britain, so placing a government seal of approval on the emerging orthodoxy of biomedicine. The novel was therefore being written in an important period of transition for medicine, when ideas of equality and inequality in health and in medical care were fast gaining ground, but were still highly contentious. The characters in the story inhabit two ideologically separate worlds, some of them respecting the norms and values of a passing epoch, whilst the others reject them and look to the future. The hero, Dr Thorne, is portrayed as a family doctor who is firmly wedded to the new era, and derives his professional authority from the claims to universal jurisdiction of the new medical science and technology. Thus in the rural village of Greshamsbury he treats everyone as an equal regardless of their social standing, much to the consternation of Lady Arabella. She, as a staunch member of the opposite camp, has more traditional views, and until Dr Thorne's arrival had only consulted with physicians from the neighbouring town.

This part of the narrative, which centres on the exchange between them, is mirrored by that involving Dr Thorne's illegitimate niece Mary, who as the heroine, is courted by and eventually marries Lady Arabella's son. The prospect of such a match fills Lady Arabella with horror, whereas Dr Thorne regards Mary as the equal of any aristocrat. What divides them is whether the biological and social uncertainty arising from her illegitimate birth is to count. For Lady Arabella they are everything, but for Dr Thorne very little. So the two strands of the story are complementary, and reinforce one another in drawing the contrast between the old and new ideas about equality.

The arguments advanced so far mainly concern the meaningfulness of notions of equality in health and in medical care for all citizens, rather than their desirability as a goal to be pursued. No attempt will be made to analyse the historical reason for their becoming seen as desirable by society in general, but the fact that this was so, can be inferred from their increasing incorporation into health policy as the nineteenth century progressed. This also entailed a growing acceptance of public responsibility, which is in marked contrast with the late seventeenth century and eighteenth century, when the idea of national health as a public concern involved only a general notion of the health of the whole population in relation to the economic well-being of the country. The health and medical care of individuals were then seen as primarily a private responsibility, in which it would have been improper for public policy to intrude. The differences in perception involved the abstract health of a social body in the eighteenth century, compared with the concrete health of an individual biological body in more modern times.

Increasing State and Public Intervention

How, though, did this transition to greater public involvement come about? There were many important elements, but one which was most significant in Britain was the emergence of the early public health movement in the 1830s. This was because it was underpinned by Benthamite utilitarianism (as interpreted by Chadwick and his followers), which was reliant on the strict equality of all people. Bentham claimed to be able to compute 'the greatest happiness of the greatest number', and this depended on the egalitarian notion embodied in his felicific calculus.[8] So the practical developments in public health in the period from about 1830 to 1860 are an early instantiation of ideas of equality in relation to health. However, they mainly concerned sanitary engineering, which was implemented at a collective level, and was politically divorced from mainstream medicine, despite the involvement of a number of prominent medical practitioners such as Dr Southwood Smith. Hence at this stage public health did not engage with the individual biological body, but was an interim phase between the humoralism of the eighteenth century and its associated physiological conception of disease, and biomedicine of the later nineteenth century and its ontological conception of disease. The difference between physiological and ontological conceptions of disease concerns two opposing viewpoints. The former sees 'the origins of disease in an imbalance between the forces of nature within and outside the sick person', whereas the latter 'understands diseases to be *entities*, things that invade and are localized in parts of the body'.[9]

Nevertheless the ontological conception of disease, which was to become central to biomedicine, was developing alongside the public health movement. This can be seen in the operation of the Registrar General's Office for England and Wales which was established in 1836 for the national collection and statistical calculations of births and deaths by age and cause. It marked the transition from the idea of death as a natural event accompanied by illness, to that of death as a pathological event caused by disease. Of particular relevance for the subsequent medicalization of public health was the development of the Infant Mortality Rate (IMR) relating to deaths occurring in the first year of life.

Since the late nineteenth century, it has become regarded as the most useful measure in comparing the health of whole societies, as well as subgroups within them, most notably by social class. It is the statistic above all others which has become universally acknowledged in epidemiology and public health. As such, it has acquired an ontological status of its own, comparable in public health to that of disease in clinical medicine. So it is not surprising that although the raw data for the calculation of IMRs had been available for many years,[10] it did not come into existence as a distinct entity with its familiar modern connotations until the 1870s. As Armstrong observes:

> In 1857 the number of deaths under the age of one year were provided for the whole country and in subsequent years an annual breakdown of infant deaths by various causes was published, but it was not until 1877 that infant deaths were specifically reported as the infant mortality rate . . . It was of course possible, retrospectively, to calculate the infant mortality rate (IMR) for the years preceding 1875 so that changes in the rate in both earlier and subsequent years could be identified and compared. Yet this contemporary (and modern) emphasis on the content of the statistic should not detract from the historical significance of its form.[11]

So the use of statistics in this way only developed slowly, in parallel with the emerging assumptions that lay at the root of biomedicine and clinical practice, and both were dependent on, as well as encouraging, ideas of equality in health and in medical care.

Whilst public health was evolving, there were also developments in the public provision of medical care in the first half of the

nineteenth century, but these were mainly restricted to those who
were not seen to be equal to the population in general, but by their
nature different and marginal. For example, the insane were
increasingly provided for within county asylums, under the Acts of
1808 and 1845, although, as with public institutions more generally, these were originally optional, and universal provision did not
come till later. This contrasts with the utilitarian (and hence also
egalitarian) principle which informed the Poor Law Amendment
Act of 1834. It determined that the inmates of the workhouses
were not to be in any way advantaged in relation to the working
poor of the general population, and this included their provision of
medical care. Thus in a strict sense the indigent and the working
poor were being regarded as equals, despite the reality that a large
proportion of paupers were unequal in being chronically ill and
disabled and so deserving of additional care. It is significant
though, that this was not officially recognized until 1867 when the
Metropolitan Poor Act allowed for the provision of Poor Law
infirmaries alongside but separate from the workhouses, which
shows how the Benthamite idea of strict equality, did not give way
to the modern notion of equity – equal care for those with equal
needs[12] – until the 1860s.

Once again it can be seen how a political notion of equality only
became modified later to attain its modern meaning under the
growing influence of biomedicine. The original political assumption was that individuals are principally responsible for their own
welfare, including their health, whereas later it was acknowledged
that the chronically sick and disabled are incapable of taking
responsibility for their own health, and so will be unfairly
disadvantaged if dealt with strictly as equals. By the 1860s, this
gave legitimacy to the improved public provision of medical care,
based on the new understanding that people may be politically
equal but medically different, a more complex idea which would
have been impossible in an earlier period.

By about 1870, then, the assumptions and values associated with
biomedicine had become predominant in both clinical medicine
and public health, and were congruent with a range of other new
ideas. Most notably for this chapter, these included those concerning inequalities in health and in medical care, and were being
interpreted in a manner which still continues today. They had also
become matters of public concern. However, despite an awareness

since this time of systematic inequalities in health, the politicians, the medical profession and the public have consistently paid more attention to developing public policies for reducing inequalities in medical care than in health. The next section of this chapter will therefore be concerned with describing a variety of different ways in which this has come about, and examining the reasons for it.

Strategies for Dealing with Inequalities in Health and in Medical Care in the Modern Period

Redefinition

Public health became medicalized between the 1850s and 1870s, and several interlocking elements were involved in its transformation. There was first a change in theoretical orientation from miasmatism to contagionism, which has parallels with the transition from humoralism to biomedicine. Miasmatism holds that ill health is caused by noxious emanations arising from polluted environments, whereas contagionism presumes that there is a direct causal relationship between each particular disease and a specific factor or factors associated with it. Second was a change in professional control, from an overt association with politics and economics to that of mainstream medicine. Finally, there was also a change in the orientation of public health, from sanitary engineering to the surveillance of health and disease of populations.

So by the end of the nineteenth century public health had become recognized as the third arm within a tripartite medical structure, with an apparently clear division of public responsibility between care for health of the population (public health) and medical care (hospital medicine and general practice). This would suggest that public health should have as a central focus the emerging concerns about inequalities in health. Although to some extent this was true and has remained so ever since, public health began further to redefine its role from this time, away from issues of health and towards medical care. This came about in two important ways. First, it became involved with the management of publicly provided medical care, and as such care grew, this role grew with it. This then came to be a major part of the medical officer of health's expanding empire, reaching its height between 1929 and 1948, when the management of Poor Law infirmaries was added to his brief. Second, from the early years of the twentieth century, there were significant developments in public services relating to personal preventive care (for example, maternal and child health services and the school health service), and these were also included within public health's remit.

The problem for public health as a professional institution was that its incorporation into mainstream medicine involved a compromise which made it very difficult for the health of the population, rather than medical care, to remain its principal concern. Even to speak of the 'medicalization' of public health is to imply that medicine is not properly about the social and political issues, which were the concerns of its early founders, and are necessarily raised in considering questions of inequalities in health. Rather, it is taken for granted that being seen as part of medicine entails an acceptance of the very assumptions and values of biomedicine, particularly value-free knowledge, and a focus on disease in individuals, and this militates against any wider conception of or concern with health. So, not surprisingly, public health doctors have always had an ambiguous relationship with mainstream medicine. If health is their main focus they are not readily acceptable, but to compete for patients is intolerable to clinicians, as well as a denial of the separate role and identity of public health. The additional roles of management and personal prevention that public health adopted can be seen as an attempt to avoid these difficulties, by both reducing the emphasis on health, and being complementary to rather than competing with clinical medicine. This allowed public health to identify more clearly with biomedicine, but in doing so inevitably diminished its profile and authority in relation to inequalities in health. At the same time, through its management role, it increasingly came to be identified with concerns about inequalities in medical care.

Another aspect of these redefinitions of role was the attempt by public health doctors to raise their traditionally low status within medicine as a whole. However, this was largely unsuccessful, with these manoeuvrings serving chiefly to re-emphasize the dominance of clinical medicine. This failure to command status within medicine has then served to reduce the impact of the work on inequalities in health that public health has continued to produce.

Suppression

In the inter-war years, the main concern of those involved with health and medical care was how best to organize and deliver medical services for the population as a whole. In retrospect, this can be seen as a period of public policy debate which culminated in the setting up of the NHS in 1948, and issues of inequality in medical care were central to this debate.

In contrast, those concerns that were frequently raised during the Depression of the 1930s, about the nation's health and especially about inequalities in health, were consistently denied by the government, and Webster has argued:

> Notwithstanding their solid features, founded on the fine Victorian tradition of public health reporting, the inter-war Annual Reports [of Government] bear the unmistakable imprint of complacency. These reports were essentially reports of progress, and nothing was allowed to detract from this image. There was no absence of criticism or of appeals for greater effort, but never were deficiencies in the record systematically explored. Thus the Reports risked becoming a means whereby a body of unquestionably accurate data was manipulated by the medical bureaucracy to defend the status quo.[13]

What was principally obscured, as Webster goes on to show, was that although average IMRs for England and Wales did not worsen in the inter-war years, the long-term downward trend was adversely affected. Also this average rate concealed very large variations between geographical regions, areas and districts, and these were closely correlated with economic and social conditions. But this evidence of inequalities in health associated with poverty and unemployment was consistently ignored.

Much of the raw data from which these government reports were derived came from the annual reports of medical officers of health which were compiled for every local authority as a statutory obligation, and the detail in them often contradicted this rosy picture. What is notable though is that the medical officers of health did not counter this message in any significant way. There was a notable case of frank suppression by government,[14] but more importantly public health did not have the power or will to mount a convincing challenge. Medical officers of health were both distracted with their burgeoning management role and reluctant to become engaged in an overtly political struggle which would have called into question the credibility of public health as a medical and scientifically objective discipline.

Reconciliation

Implicit in the creation of the NHS was a very widely held notion that by providing the best available care for all medical needs, not only would care for each individual patient be maximized, but the health of the population and also inequalities in health would improve automatically. It was therefore assumed that given that the sanitary reforms of the nineteenth century were in place, further improvements in health were largely a function of improvements in medical care. This then allowed for a reconciliation between the goals of correcting inequalities in medical care and in health, without having to pay attention to the latter. Thus, as Lawrence notes, the Ministry of Health, which was established in 1919, 'was not a ministry of health at all, it was a ministry of clinical medicine',[15] mainly concerned with improving and developing medical care. This principally meant medical treatment, but was also to be complemented by personal preventive medicine which the first chief medical officer to the ministry, Sir George Newman, described in 1931 as deriving from the knowledge, provided by laboratory scientists, clinicians and epidemiologists, which if followed would lead to a healthy life.[16]

So clinical science was seen as pointing to the future not only for medical care, but also for public policy on health, and at the same time the older notions of health and public health's role in promoting it were being sidelined. A significant expression of this thinking can be seen in the way in which Bevan devised the structure of the NHS. He decided to organize medical care on a national basis because he was concerned to rectify historic inequalities of provision between different geographical areas, but left public health within the control of local authorities, and so to the vagaries of local interpretation and funding. This suggests that Bevan was also influenced by the thesis of reconciliation, and so believing that the NHS would deal simultaneously with inequalities in health and in medical care, saw no need to bring public health activities under central control.

A further implication of this reasoning was that public responsibility for both health and medical care was increased to a degree never seen previously. Conversely private responsibility was reduced to no more than a personal duty to follow medical orders, with regard to both treatment and prevention. The prevalence and strength of this understanding at the time is well illustrated by Talcott Parsons's original description of the 'sick role' in 1951,[17] and the positivist manner in which it was interpreted, as a fixed concept within the social order. He described how he thought social stability was maintained through the interaction of doctors and patients. He suggested that when individuals became accepted as patients by doctors, they gained two benefits (being exempt from their normal social role and not being held responsible for their illness), but at the same time were expected to fulfil two obligations (wanting to get well and cooperating with medical advice in attempting to do so).

Re-emergence
For some twenty years after the NHS was set up in 1948, questions about inequalities in health and in medical care did not feature prominently on the political agenda. There was a considerable degree of political consensus during this post-war period, particularly concerning the NHS, about which there was a general feeling of national pride and satisfaction. However, by the 1960s this spell of relative calm had come to an end, with all aspects of life, including medicine and the NHS, undergoing re-examination. The reconciliation thesis, described in the last section, began to be seriously questioned, so reopening issues about both inequalities in health and in medical care.

Despite the beliefs of Bevan and the other founders of the NHS, inequality in the provision of medical care continued to persist in the 1950s and 1960s, and two developments will be described which illustrate the way the issue resurfaced politically. The first relates to Tudor Hart's famous characterization of the 'inverse care law', which was published in 1971, and held that those with most medical needs tend on average to receive the least medical care.[18] This is both because of a maldistribution of services in relation to need, and also because those with greater needs, who are mainly in the lower social classes, are less able to access services. The second development concerns the poor standard and level of services in long-stay hospitals for the chronically sick, when compared with services for the acutely ill. This came to attention following a series of scandals in such hospitals, the first being that at Ely hospital, the report on which was made public in 1969.[19] These services for the chronically ill became known as the 'Cinderella' services.

In subsequent years, attempts were made by government to address both these issues. For example, in the 1970s a Resource Allocation Working Party (RAWP)[20] was set up which applied a formula aimed at bringing about the geographical redistribution of resources in relation to medical need, and so, taken overall, from richer to poorer areas of the country. Also the 'Cinderella' services were designated as priority services, as part of a policy commitment to redirect funding positively for their improvement.

At the same time, work that had been going on for some years on the health of the population and inequalities in health also received recognition. McKeown's thesis, developed in a book entitled *The Role of Medicine*, gained particular prominence. It was first published in 1976, and in an expanded version in 1979.[21] It claimed that the historical increase in population in Britain resulting from improvement in health had principally been the result of improvements in socio-economic conditions, mediated largely via better nutrition. Public health interventions were considered of secondary importance, and most significantly, it was maintained that medical care had hardly influenced the health of the population at all. Whilst some aspects of McKeown's thesis have been challenged,[22] the relatively small effect that medical services have on population health is now generally accepted. Therefore, however much medical care and its distribution in relation to need is improved, this cannot be expected to bring about major improvements in health or reductions of inequalities in health. Thus, in theory at least, the reconciliation thesis had been overturned. It might then have been thought that the scene was set for a renewal and redirection of public policy in relation to inequalities in health that did not rely on medical care. However, with an incoming Conservative government in 1979, this was not to be.

Denial

In 1980 the Black Report on *Inequalities in Health*,[23] which had been commissioned by a Labour government in 1977, was completed and presented to the new Conservative government. It brought together a great deal of evidence and concluded that socio-economic factors were the main determinants of inequalities in health. The initial government response was to sideline the report by making available only a very limited number of copies with the least publicity possible. However, this measure backfired, leading to it becoming more celebrated than it might otherwise have been, and to the appearance of a paperback version in 1982.[24] The government's response should not be interpreted as simply a straightforward attempt at suppression, though, as the following passage from the secretary of state's foreword to the report shows:

> It will come as a disappointment to many that over long periods since the inception of the NHS there is generally little sign of health inequalities in Britain actually diminishing and, in some cases, they may be increasing. It will be seen that the Group has reached the view that the causes of health inequalities are so deep rooted that only a major and wide-ranging programme of public expenditure is capable of altering the pattern.
>
> I must make it clear that additional expenditure on the scale which could result from the report's recommendations – the amount involved could be upward of £2 billion a year – is quite unrealistic in present or any foreseeable economic circumstances, quite apart from any judgement that may be formed of the effectiveness of such expenditure in dealing with the problems identified.[25]

What this suggests is an awareness of the failure of the reconciliation thesis, and a redefinition of the government's responsibility by way of response. Essentially, medical care (mainly provided by the NHS) was being seen as a continuing public responsibility, but health was in future to be regarded as largely a private responsibility. This was a very significant retreat from the earlier political consensus, and is clearly demonstrated in the development of health policy in the 1980s. Most notable was the evolution of health promotion, and its displacement of the previous concept of health education. Ideas about health education had been derived from the understanding that government had a responsibility both to supply information and to make available the appropriate means for people to live healthy lives. The individual's responsibility was then mainly to comply with the advice given. Health promotion, on the other hand, involves the restriction of government responsibility to making information available to people in order that they can make their own choices and so take responsibility for them. Hence the

Conservative government in their response to the Black Report can be seen to be starting to articulate a new ideological position, in which inequalities in health may be unfortunate, but are no longer viewed as a public responsibility.

Contradiction

A Labour government took office in 1997 with the declared intention of re-establishing a public commitment and responsibility for inequalities in health, as well as continuing the traditional commitment to reducing inequalities in medical care through renewed attention to the NHS. It therefore commissioned the Acheson Report, which was published in 1998[26] and was essentially an updating of the Black Report, echoing its main findings. It revealed that the gap in health inequalities had not only persisted in the 1980s and 1990s but had widened, and it was considered that differences in material circumstances were the major cause.

The problem for the government in responding to this was that it uncovered a contradiction at the heart of its strategy for health policy development, which started in the customary way with a pledge to provide more money for the NHS. Crucially, though, it was proposed that this should not come from increased taxation, but from the creation of more national wealth. This was in line with a general policy aimed at improving public services from economic growth. However, the engine for such growth was dependent on market competition, which was an extension of the earlier Conservative policy of the 1980s and 1990s. Now it was just these policies which had already led to a widening of inequalities in wealth, and which the Acheson Report had identified as the main cause of the increases in inequalities in health. It would seem then that Labour's policy for reducing inequalities in medical care, by more careful targeting of those with the greatest medical need,[27] would inevitably lead to continuing or even growing differentials in inequalities in health, if financed through economic growth derived from market competition. So by placing the primary emphasis on improving medical care through material growth, the government's commitment to improving health and especially inequalities in health would seem to be compromised. Once again, reducing inequalities in health appears to have been given a higher public priority, but this is likely to prove empty in practice.

New theoretical insights have recently emerged concerning the relationship between inequalities in wealth and inequalities in health, and have been demonstrated by Wilkinson to hold across many societies.[28] Of particular relevance for this chapter has been the reappraisal of the long-held assumption that material factors are the principal cause of inequalities in health, and that increasing wealth equates directly with better health. The new evidence suggests that whilst a certain basic level of material wealth is clearly essential to health, once this is exceeded other factors are also important. This has been shown by the fact that above this level, those countries with relatively small inequalities in wealth are healthier than those where the converse is true. The reasons for this are the subject of ongoing debate, and a great deal of theoretical work remains to be done. However, what is not in doubt is that a different type of explanation is required:

> A theory is needed which unifies the causes of the health inequalities related to social hierarchy with the effects of income inequality on national mortality rates. At its centre are likely to be factors affecting how hierarchical the hierarchy is, the depths of material insecurity and social exclusion which societies tolerate, and the direct and indirect psychosocial affects of social stratification.
>
> One reason why greater income equality is associated with better health seems to be that it tends to improve social cohesion and reduce the social divisions. Qualitative and quantitative evidence suggest that more egalitarian societies are more cohesive.[29]

What seems clear from this is that current government policy is likely to lead to less social cohesion, as it did in the 1980s and early 1990s, and this will have a negative impact on health. Whatever other policies the government puts in place in an attempt to improve inequalities in health will then tend to be undermined whilst inequalities in wealth persist or widen. So until there is a recognition of this contradiction and a willingness to make more radical changes, reductions in inequalities in health will not have been given genuine priority.

What is required is a new understanding of the relationship between wealth and health, which is reflected in a different conception of the goals of policies for health and medical care and the relationship between them. Without this, a focus on inequalities in medical care, and a particular way of tackling them, will continue in reality to displace concerns about inequalities in health.

Conclusion

Addressing inequalities in health has always taken second place to considerations of inequalities in medical care, ever since they both entered the policy arena in the nineteenth century. Redressing this will continue to be problematic whilst the ideological values relating to material wealth, a positivist conception of science and individualism persist, both generally and particularly as they are expressed in biomedicine. There is a resonance between the dominant interpretation of material factors as the principal and direct cause of the health of populations, and the centrality of an ontological account of disease within medicine and health care. Refocusing on inequalities in health will therefore require simul-taneous attention to both these issues, and this will entail the inclusion of psychosocial factors, interpreted subjectively, to be integrated with material factors, so as to produce a fresh under-standing of how they influence health.

In doing this, the conceptualization of health will itself become modified towards a more Hygeian notion of health as wholeness, and away from the current Asclepian notion that views health negatively as the absence of disease and disability. This is not, though, a wholesale rejection of either the role of material factors in relation to health or of Asclepian accounts of health. Rather, it is a plea for a transformation which involves a rebalancing of concepts of health and a reinterpretation of how best to provide medical care. Scientific rationalism and materialism on their own will not resolve the problem of inequalities in medical care any more than those of inequalities in health, and only by redefining them in a way which is more symmetrical will it be possible to develop viable and enduring solutions.

Notes

[1] Porter, D. (1999), *Health, Civilization and the State* (London, Routledge), p. 66.

[2] Ibid., p. 57.

[3] Lawrence, C. (1994), *Medicine in the Making of Modern Britain, 1700–1920* (London, Routledge), p. 62.

[4] Floud, R., Wachter, K. and Gregory, A. (1990), *Height, Health and History* (Cambridge, Cambridge University Press).

[5] It has been suggested that the terms 'higher' (or upper) and 'lower' class may originally have been a literal description of the differences in height involved.

[6] An account is given of a Mr Wakefield who in 1658 turned to the local 'Horse-Smithe' for advice and treatment in Porter, D. and Porter, R. (1989), *Patient's Progress* (Cambridge, Polity Press), p. 29.

[7] Trollope, A. (1959), *Dr Thorne* (Cambridge, MA, Riverside Press; first published in 1858).

[8] These ideas were developed in Bentham, J. (1879), *An Introduction to the Principles of Morals and Legislation* (Oxford, Clarendon Press; first printed in 1780 and published in 1789 and as a new edition in 1823).

[9] Cassell, E. J. (1991), *The Nature of Suffering and the Goals of Medicine* (New York and London, Oxford University Press), p. 4.

[10] Before national registration was introduced, births, marriages and deaths had been recorded locally in parish registers for several centuries.

[11] Armstrong, D. (1986), 'The invention of infant mortality', *Sociology of Health and Illness*, 8, 211–32 (212).

[12] This idea derives from Aristotle's formal principle of justice or equality (in the *Nicomachean Ethics*) according to which equals should be treated equally and unequals unequally in proportion to relevant inequalities.

[13] Webster, C. (1982), 'Healthy or hungry thirties?', *History Workshop Journal*, 13, 110–29 (112)

[14] McGonigle, G. C. M. and Kirby, J. (1936), *Poverty and Public Health* (London, Gollancz).

[15] Lawrence, *Medicine in the Making of Modern Britain*, p. 82.

[16] Newman, G. (1931), *Health and Social Evaluation* (London, George Allen and Unwin).

[17] Parsons, T. (1951), *The Social System* (Glencoe, IL, Free Press).

[18] Hart, J. T. (1971), 'The inverse care law', *Lancet*, 1, 405–12.

[19] *Report of the Committee of Inquiry into Allegations of Ill-Treatment of Patients and Other Irregularities at the Ely Hospital, Cardiff* (1969), Cmnd. 3975 (London, HMSO).

[20] DHSS (1976), Report of the Resource Allocation Working Party, *Sharing Resources for Health in England* (London, HMSO).

[21] McKeown, T. (1979), *The Role of Medicine* (Oxford, Blackwell).

[22] One challenge to McKeown's thesis is based on the grounds that the public health movement has had a significant influence on the nation's health. See for example Szreter, S. (1988), 'The importance of social interaction in Britain's mortality decline c. 1850–1914: a re-interpretation of the role of public health', *Social History of Medicine*, 1, 1–37. Another important question is whether pursuing prevention rather than cure is necessarily a good thing. See for example Skrabanek, P. (1994), *The Death of Humane Medicine* (London, The Social Affairs Unit).

[23] DHSS (1980), unpublished report of a research working group, 'Inequalities in Health'.

[24] Townsend, P. and Davidson, N. (eds) (1982), *Inequalities in Health: The Black Report* (Harmondsworth, Penguin).

[25] DHSS *Inequalities*, Foreword.

[26] Acheson, D. (1998), *Independent Inquiry into Inequalities in Health* (London, HMSO).

[27] This can be seen in the government's support for evidence-based practice, and the setting-up of the National Institute for Clinical Excellence (NICE).

[28] Wilkinson, R.G. (1996), *Unhealthy Societies* (London, Routledge).

[29] Wilkinson, R. G. (1997), 'Health inequalities: relative or absolute material standards?', *British Medical Journal*, 314, 591–5 (593).

Index